Social Action in Group Work

The *Social Work with Groups* series

Social Action in Group Work

Abe Vinik
Morris Levin
Editors

The Haworth Press, Inc.
New York • London • Sydney

Social Action in Group Work has also been published as *Social Work with Groups*, Volume 14, Numbers 3/4 1991.

The Haworth Press, Inc. 10 Alice Street, Binghamton, NY 13904-1580
EUROSPAN/Haworth, 3 Henrietta Street, London WC2E 8LU England
ASTAM/Haworth, 162-168 Parramatta Road, Stanmore, Sydney, N.S.W. 2048 Australia

Library of Congress Cataloging-in-Publication Data

Social action in group work / Abe Vinik, Morris Levin, editors.
    p. cm.
    "Also . . . published as Social work with groups, volume 14, numbers 3/4, 1991" — T.p. verso.
    ISBN 1-56024-211-6 (alk. paper). — ISBN 1-56024-212-4 (pbk.: alk. paper)
    1. Social group work. 2. Social action. I. Vinik, Abe. II. Levin, Morris.
HV45.S613 1992
361.4 — dc20
                                                    91-39986
                                                      CIP

Social Action in Group Work

CONTENTS

ALL HAWORTH BOOKS & JOURNALS
ARE PRINTED ON CERTIFIED
ACID-FREE PAPER

ABOUT THE EDITORS

Abe Vinik and **Morris Levin** have shared more than forty years of professional practice together as colleagues, collaborators and friends. Both studied social group work with Grace Coyle at Case-Western Reserve University in the 1940's and pursued their careers in neighborhood based agencies, retiring in the 1980's as executive directors with the United Jewish Community Centers in the San Francisco Metropolitan Area and the Jewish Community Centers of Chicago. Each has taught group process at the University of Chicago and other schools of social work in the U.S. They have held board leadership positions in NASW and other professional organizations and institutions, written extensively—with primary focus on group work theory, board and staff development, agency planning and administration, and served as consultants for the State Department in Europe and Israel. Since their retirement they have concentrated their consultation to local and national organizations in the areas of executive development, evaluation of agency structures and programs, and continuing education for professional staff.

Preface

The health and vitality of the group work sector of the profession of social work is embodied in this volume on *Social Action in Group Work*. It was conceived as a much needed special issue of the journal *Social Work With Groups*. The Co-Editors of the journal, the late Beulah Rothman and myself, knew that the subject was a worthy one when we invited Abe Vinik and Morris Levin to work on it, but the intellectual process and the outcome were beyond expectation. Guest Editors Vinik and Levin are to be honored for the manner in which they have engaged many distinguished social group work professionals in exploring the subject. A new level of consideration of the commitment to social change and participatory democracy that is inherent in social work's societal mission is opened up for the profession. This is a worthy volume to be presented not only as a double issue of the volume but also to be included in the Haworth *Social Work With Groups* Series, and thus to be available as a text for the education of social workers and the dissemination of professional knowledge. Vinik and Levin present a timely challenge for an ongoing discourse on social action in this social group work journal and in all professional social work literature during the treacherous decade that is closing the twentieth century.

In the immediate past issue of *Social Work With Groups*, Volume XIV (2) Summer 1991, conceptual and theoretical discussions of empowerment as a significant social work objective word presented and illustrated. Of the three levels of empowerment—individual, interpersonal and political—political empowerment seemed the most unlikely to be actualized in the various practice papers presented in that issue. In the Editorial the question was asked: "Why?" Is it present but not reported? In the life of a group is the progression from personal through interpersonal to political empowerment an epigenetic process? Does the key to the realization of political empowerment in the group rest with the committment of the worker?

Considering political empowerment and social action as closely related concepts, several categories of suggestions or clues for answering such questions are to be found in the manuscripts presented in this serial issue under the guest editorship of Vinik and Levin.

1. Some *populations,* e.g., groups of women, may be particularly ready and eager for social action.
2. Some *theoretical or philosophical perspectives* for group work are highly suggestive and productive of empowerment of members, e.g., liberation theology and conscietization.
3. Some *aspects of a worker's behavior and attributes* facilitate an outcome of empowerment in the group, e.g., equality in the professional stance of the worker.
4. Some *professional skills* which encourage an empowerment outcome can be identified.

Again Vinik and Levin are to be thanked for uncovering such a wealth of professional material to foster social action and political empowerment in group work practice and in research.

With this issue of *Social Work With Groups* — and with this Editorial — the era of the original and present co-editorship is drawn to a close. Beulah Rothman and I had decided early in the fateful year of her illness and death that we were ready to yield to others the excitement of editing the social group work journal. In April of 1990 we wrote to Bill Cohen, Publisher of The Haworth Press, Inc., resigning as Co-Editors and proposing persons to replace us. Our suggestions were graciously accepted and with the completion of this issue, Number 3/4 of Volume 14, our responsibilities are terminated.

The new Editors are Roselle Kurland, Professor of Social Group Work at Hunter School of Social Work, and Andrew Malekoff, Coordinator of the Suburban Family Life Center and the Alcohol Treatment and Prevention Services at the North Shore Child and Family Guidance Center. Volume 15 (1992) is being prepared by them in their new roles.

When we were asked in 1976 to co-edit a journal on groups in social work, a form of social work service traditionally present at that time but theoretically faded and fragmented, the perspective for such a journal was carefully weighed. It was to be dedicated to a holistic view of social group work, and of the social work profession. The title of the journal, *Social Work With Groups*, was selected to communicate the breadth of conception of the place of the small group in a multi-functional social work profession. The subtitle stated the point of view more explicitly—"A Journal of Community and Clinical Practice." The original Editorial Policy Statement for *Social Work With Groups*, written by these Co-Editors at the inception of the journal fourteen years ago is presented again for its readers, old and new.

EDITORIAL POLICY STATEMENT

There is no profession that places a greater value on the individual in his/her social context than does the profession of social work. For most people the social context becomes manageable and definable through the small group. Now more than ever, in an alienating and anomic work, there is the necessity for the human group to carry its functions: the linking of individuals with each other as they struggle to achieve fullness and the production morale, leadership, and cooperation, the bonding ingredients for a viable society.

During the past two decades as the profession has been strengthening its central unity it has seemed that the unique social work contribution to understanding and working with the small group is being lost. It is our conviction, to the contrary, that in this period of time social work has been quietly developing a new and mature identity in relation to group practice. This journal hopes to set forth that new identity, incorporating the vitality of our history with the richness and complexity of the psychosocial orientation of our profession. It is no longer only the group workers in the social work profession who carry the passion for the human group and the commitment to its use in relation to social work purposes, but the profession itself.

It is the intent of *Social Work With Groups* to serve as a vehicle of communication for the several sectors of our profession wherein the small group heritage and the building of knowledge and skills of group practice are embodied. There are those who represent the early group work tradition from the community and neighborhood centers with focus on socialization in groups and the contribution of the healthy group to social betterment. There are those who represent the clinical tradition with focus on the therapeutic value of the small group and on the family as a small group. There are those who represent the community and planning tradition with focus on mobilizing and developing social resources and neighborhoods through the energies of task groups. Finally, there are those who represent administration and social policy with focus on welding together a humanizing service system through the collective efforts of staff and community groups. It is to the enrichment and dissemination of these professional labors that this journal of group work theory and practice is dedicated.

In rereading this Statement there is experienced a sense of pride in the perspective, the direction and the achievement. In addition there is the related timeliness of our final issue represented by this volume on *Social Action in Group Work.*

For the retiring co-editors of *Social Work With Groups* the journal was a mission! The power of healthy group life for the society, for individual growth and well-being, and as a means of social work helping was the committment. It remained so throughout Beulah Rothman's life and continues in mine. This has been shared by the members of the journal's Advisory Board during these fourteen years and I believe by you, its readers. The work to be done in such an endeavor can not ever be complete, so may it go on with new inspiration and vitality in *Social Work With Groups,* in the literature of social group work and of the social work profession!

Catherine P. Papell
Co-Editor

Acknowledgements

Many thanks are due from the editors and authors to those whose feedback helped mold the papers finally selected for inclusion in this volume.

The following individuals served as the Editorial Review Board for Social Action in Group Work:

Mark G. Battle	Eve Lodge
Margaret Berry	Sanford Solender
Richard J. Estes	Harry Specht
Mitchell I. Ginsberg	Herman Stein
Audreye E. Johnson	Alvin Zander

xv

Introduction

Abe Vinik
Morris Levin

This special volume was inspired in the aftermath of the centennial celebration of Jane Addams' founding of Hull House. For Catherine Papell and the late Beulah Rothman, Co-Editors of *Social Work with Groups* since its founding in 1978, it seemed an appropriate theme for the work to be produced under their direction. They shared a growing unease about the neglect, and even subversion, of societal change as a purpose of social work, and in particular, of social group work. They hoped their publication would contribute to a professional renewal of group work's early commitments, with new insights, knowledge, methods, and skills to make social action-oriented practice more effective and pervasive.

For this volume a series of questions were raised and prospective authors invited to address them. Among these questions: How significant a role did social action play in the origins of work with groups and social group work? What were the philosophies and purposes from which it originated? What were its scope and effectiveness, its successes and failure? Why? What influenced the decline and/or reemergence of social action in group work? What can and should be done to influence existing trends? What are the sources to which social group workers can look to nourish their commitment to social change?

Responses, suggestive and exciting, came quickly and in greater number than anticipated. Interested authors proposed some answers and posed new issues offering sufficient challenge to stimulate further thinking, exploring and testing. Together the writers of these collected papers leave the reader with the need to determine how firm is the base of democratic participation and social justice on which to build. What do such contemporary issues as consciousness raising, feminist theory and liberation theology have in common with social groupwork, and can they be integrated with discrete contributions to social action practice? And what of empowerment and advocacy in social work with groups?

IDEAS OF SOCIAL ACTION (HISTORY AND REALITY)

Fourteen papers are presented in three sections, each with its own focus although the concepts, theories and models overlap. The first, Ideas of Social Action, ranges from Shapiro's examination of the history of social action in group work, to Staub-Bernasconi's proposal for an integrated global framework for social work organization, education and practice from a West European perspective. Wood and Middleman locate the place of advocacy and social action in their structural model of practice. Lewis identifies the strengths and weaknesses of feminist theory and liberation theology and their contribution to a more realistic understanding by social workers of the individual's relation to society. Finally, Garvin deals with existing impediments to social action practice, suggesting how these might begin to be overcome.

There has been agreement among social group work theorists and educators that social group work practice can and should lead to action. Shapiro concludes that "there has been an 'ebb and flow' in the 'centrality' of social action activity over the years." This comes as no surprise. Since 1930 we have experienced a major depression, four wars, four political assassinations, a sensitization to the real extent of poverty, racial and ethnic conflict, and other serious dislocations and disruptions.

These realities compel us to assess our heightened awareness of societal problems through the perspective of the current theoretical and applied social science knowledge, and through our collective practice wisdom joined with our best intuitions.

The authors agree that individual problems are too often rooted in social structures which do not afford the opportunity for evenhanded results. In order to identify the problem source it is necessary to locate it in the social structure and to understand how the functions of a social structure work.

Acknowledging the influence of Talcott Parsons' functional social theory in Western (American) social work and social welfare thought, Staub-Bernasconi notes, "There should be a challenge to the dominating functional perspective." She calls for and suggests the outline for an evolutionary general systems social theory as an alternative. A study of social work curricula to assess this appraisal would be rewarding.

ADVOCACY AND EMPOWERMENT

In section II Cox defines empowerment practice and gives case examples of work with disadvantaged adults and elderly women. Wood and Middleman outline steps in carrying out advocacy. Keenan and Pinkerton, Breton, and Mullender and Ward pursue the subject further in their analyses of practice examples with severely disadvantaged youth (beyond the North American experience). Since advocacy and empowerment are orientations usually found under agency or organizational auspices, Taylor's exploration of the use of agency structure to support and enhance such practice adds a usually neglected dimension for consideration.

Wood and Middleman suggest a method for identifying the need for advocacy in the scope and severity of the problem. One way of working toward problem resolution is to identify the solution which would evoke the "least contest." Breton makes the same point by stressing the need for partnership among all sectors involved in the attempt at problem resolution.

The grim demographics which introduce empowerment practice in Northern Ireland magnify the fine line between gnawing, constant hurt and alienation. Keenan and Pinkerton's fine case example as well as Mullender and Ward's work in England illustrate various social group work approaches towards overcoming the feelings and consequences of powerlessness.

PRINCIPLES AND PRACTICE

The third section explores the application of social group work to womens' groups (Home), inter-ethnic conflict (Norman), a group of homeless men and women (Sachs), and in community organization (Mondros and Berman-Rossi). Whether with a "traditional" or "radical" orientation, these papers call for further reflection on the role of the worker and her/his relationship to group process, to the individual in the group, and to social action as group program.

Lewis, Home and Cox cite feminist theory and suggest that it can make group life more effective. Women, they say, are process oriented, patient and ready to share leadership and resources. Lewis and Sachs propose that liberation theology enhances group work practice when groups can "insist upon participation in the economic and political spheres of life by those most vulnerable to its injustices." The authors hold that both liberation theology and feminist theory together support the basic social goals of social work — democratic participation and social justice.

CONCLUSION

We need, the authors say, a more sensitive practice, a more empowerment oriented practice, more advocacy by the worker and by the group, and by both with equal responsibility. We need an ability to work with systems and their structures, and a professional role in creating partnerships. What we do not need, they maintain, is the professional as expert who focuses only on content and outcome. We need a relationship of equality between group members and group workers.

There seems to be an assumption that social group work practice today is, in fact, content-driven and that a correction is in order. The underlying tension which exists between the desire for action (social action) and the desire for process in group life is inevitable. Both are essential requirements for effective empowerment practice. Their interaction is the catalyst for social action. Groups and their members represent more than objects of potential power. When the group purpose — as process — unfolds, this very tension can provide the energy for its own release and resolution. The tension between content and process is then experienced, known, explained, and transformed into group action.

These papers may serve the pursuit of dialogue among authors and readers toward the development of theory, method, and most of all, practice for social change that our time so desperately needs. Such an outcome would indeed be a most deserved tribute to Catherine Papell and memorial to Beulah Rothman for their affirmation of the distinctiveness of social group work purposes, method, and skill.

Social Action, the Group and Society

Ben Zion Shapiro

SUMMARY. There is a longstanding commitment to social action in Group Work. This can be traced back to the work of Jane Addams and Grace Coyle and many others with whom they worked and shared ideas.

However, as we follow the history of Group Work we find a shift in the meaning of social action. The role of groups in society has changed from that of instrument for social change to that of training ground for democracy.

The more recent writing of Lee, Breton, Lewis and others suggests the possibility of restoring the centrality of groups to social action in the context of new social realities and contemporary thinking about society and the state.

Group workers have never tired of reminding their colleagues that the commitment to social action goes back to the origins of the profession and the roots of social work practice with groups. Judith Lee is eloquent in her plea: "Return home and reaffirm our heri-

Ben Zion Shapiro, PhD, is on the faculty of Social Work, University of Toronto, 246 Bloor St. West, Toronto, Ontario, M5S 1A1, Canada.

tage. . . . Jane Addams won't you please come home?" (1987, pp. 3, 15)

As the political pendulum swung between eras of conservatism and liberalism, and professional theory shifted between therapy and social change, the advocates of social action moved back and forth between the mainstream and the radical fringe of the profession.

Social action advocates saw themselves as professionally responsible to help group members become aware of their competence and power to participate in the processes of social change. Early on, education for responsible citizenship was a goal of social work with groups. Social action as a group program activity was also a vehicle for learning and personal development.

The group has been recognized as a social microcosm in which its members can be helped to become participants and leaders in social action through experience with the group process and through engaging in social action processes in the group's immediate social environment.

Can the conceptualization of the group as microcosm of society go beyond the meanings currently available: that the group provides a useful training ground for democracy; that social relations in the broader social structure influence interpersonal relations within the group; and, that the group mediates between individuals and their social environment?

Can social action be integrated in group work? Does the group have a role to play as part of the social structure? Is there a practice theory of group work that is "political" in the sense that it focuses on the role and power of groups in society?

A conception of practice which sees groups as instruments for social change was close to the thinking of some early leaders in group work, though it seems to have been side-tracked along the way.

EARLY WRITERS ON SOCIAL ACTION IN GROUP WORK

The pioneers in social work with groups shared a concern for the development of a democratic society within the United States and internationally. Their work can be traced in the association between

Jane Addams and John Dewey in Chicago in the 1890's and in a more organized affiliation among Dewey, Mary Parker Follett, Eduard Lindeman, Grace Coyle and others in a group called The Inquiry in the 1920's and early 1930's.

A distinctive aspect of their ideas was an emphasis on the role of groups and voluntary associations in a pluralistic society. Groups would provide an arena within which individual interests and differences might be "socialized" (to use Jane Addams' term) and mediated. A democratic state would provide the instrumentality for group differences to be expressed, contributed for the common good, and integrated.

The work of John Dewey is seminal in this respect. Dewey's philosophy of education (1900) was deeply rooted in a view of democratic society in which "the school itself shall be made a genuine form of active community life, instead of a place set apart in which to learn lessons" (p. 22). Dewey saw the future of democracy in voluntary association. Dewey's work, from 1894 to 1904, coincided with that of Jane Addams while at the University of Chicago, and then with the group eventually associated in The Inquiry.

Two years after Dewey, Jane Addams presented her theory of education (1902), and the "striking parallels" between the two have been pointed out (Scott, 1964, p. lvi).

Addams wrote, "the educational activities of a Settlement, as well as its philanthropic, civic, and social undertakings, are but differing manifestations of the attempt to socialize democracy, as is the very existence of the Settlement itself" (1910, p. 453). Just as Dewey saw the educational system as a part of, rather than apart from society, she saw the Settlement and its programs for persons of all ages and walks of life having a direct impact on the social process.

Charles Horton Cooley called Jane Addams, "one of the most searching and yet hopeful critics of our times" (1909, p. 350). With Addams, he saw the primacy of group life as a basic social fact to be understood and taken into account in formulating a theory of democracy and the state.

Mary Parker Follett was acknowledged for her influence on many subsequent theorists in group work, administration, and political theory. She developed "the group principle" as a key element in her theory of the "new" democratic state and saw "group organization, both the neighbourhood and the occupational group," as "democracy's method" in opposition to the "crowd philosophy."

> Group organization will create the new world we are now blindly feeling after, for creative force comes from the group, creative power is evolved through the activity of the group. (1920, p. 3)

Her ideas were more specific than those of Dewey in terms of the role of groups and clearly built on those of Cooley.

Eduard Lindeman was associated with Mary Parker Follett and shared many of her ideas in relation to the role of groups in society and the state. "He wanted to understand better how one could help communities determine their own fate and how experts and citizens could work together" (Konopka, 1958). He developed his analysis with a greater emphasis on the integration of understanding and action within a value framework (1924).

R.M. MacIver, a political economist and, for a time, Director of the School of Social Service at the University of Toronto, emphasized a view of the state as association, rather than as institution, incorporating similar ideas to those of Follett, and acknowledged her work (1926).

The organization called "The Inquiry," working between 1923 and 1933, brought Dewey, Follett, and MacIver, as well as Harrison S. Elliott of the YMCA and Alfred D. Sheffield of Wellesley College together with Coyle, Lindeman, Ada Sheffield, and other social workers.

> It is this great power of the small group process that these leaders sought to harness for social goals and social betterment in a democratic, pluralistic, just society. . . . Follett, Lindeman, and Lasker, in particular, were interested in a worldwide dissemination of these ideas and in the use of group work for peaceful, communal, and democratic international relations. (Siporin, 1986)

The Inquiry went beyond social analysis, articulating an approach that emphasized harnessing group processes for purposes of social action. The "discussion method" was seen as "integrating and transforming individual interests, goals, and wills into common ones. It provides a way of arriving at necessary group decisions as a basis for collective problem-solving action and for group cohesion and self-government" (Siporin, 1986, p. 41).

More than its contribution to a social theory of groups and group methods, the Inquiry served as a forum for sharing ideas about groups and social action.

Grace Coyle was pivotal in translating the work of many of these social theorists for social workers and group workers in particular. Her doctoral dissertation at Columbia was done under the supervision of MacIver and was the basis of her first major publication. In it she affirmed that "although often in partial and inadequate form, every group relationship helps to establish that devotion of the self to super-personal ends upon which rests the hope of democratic society" (1930, p. 6). Coyle tied her analysis of social processes in groups and associations into an appreciation of their role in the broader society.

She juxtaposed Group Work with Social Change, presenting it as an experience in collective living, encouraging cultural activities which have significant social functions essential for the "cohesive, unified and enriched society which we desire," which taps the "great molten stream of social discontent and social injustice underlying present conditions," and provides direct education on social questions and social action.

1. In the first place, (the group worker) can encourage and develop social interests within his own groups. This takes skill and insight but it can be done. This will often culminate in the group participating in social action as it sees fit. The educational process in this line cannot stop short of experience in social action if it is to be effective.
2. He can help members of this agency, as they mature, to find their place in the organized life of the community, in those social action groups through which their collective interests are finding expression.
3. He can see that provision is made in the agency for the free discussion of the basic economic and social conflicts which are

so crucial to any adequate solution of the present crisis. (1935, p. 404)

Coyle's influence on theory and education for practice in group work paralleled her own interest and activity in the realm of social action and reflected her broad social concerns. She saw herself as following in the tradition of Jane Addams (1961).

Although their vision of groups as part of the polity is not a single one, and the emphasis in their political philosophy varies, these writers saw a close connection between the social action imperative and the role of groups in society.

WHAT HAPPENED TO THE WORK OF THE EARLY WRITERS?

As social work in general became more institutionalized and professionalized, more articulated and defined, community organization and administration on one hand and case work on the other asserted their separate and distinct characteristics. Group methods found their way into administration, community organization and case work and group work ceased to have a monopoly on work with groups.

Group work faced a critical set of choices: to define itself as an eclectic set of practices ranging across the spectrum of social work concerns where the use of groups might make a contribution to the helping process—including social action; to search out for itself a delimited set of group-related models distinct from other social work methods; or, to define itself as a unique and unitary social work method. None of these choices would allow for social action to be the *central* concern of group work.

The growth of theory and research dealing with processes and dynamics in small groups led to a new emphasis on the technological aspects of using groups for social work purposes. The role of values and goals had to make room for technology.

As group work theorists increasingly studied and applied materials from the social sciences, they tended to distance themselves from political theory. As they became more interested in the personal and the interpersonal, they became less interested in theories of the state and their implications for group practice.

Indeed, political thought and democratic theory in the United States, with notable exceptions including those referred to above, has tended to be inherently inimical to a role for groups and associations in the governance of society. Individualism was a paramount value in American society long before psychoanalytic ideas captured the imagination of American social workers.

Had group workers continued their interest in political thought, they would have found that it had abandoned the group oriented concerns of Follett and Coyle. Harold Laski, the British political theorist who had been of great interest to Grace Coyle, changed his perspective from group oriented pluralism to a Marxist frame of reference, and MacIver moved to an internationalist "macro" orientation and comparative political theory.

In many respects, the work of Addams, Lindeman and Coyle is reflected in, and continued by, the "Social Goals Model" of group work as articulated by Papell and Rothman, who also identify it with the work of Kaiser, Phillips, Konopka, Cohen, Miller, Ginsberg, Wilson, and Klein (1966, pp. 67-68). They see this model as offering an approach in which every group possesses "a potential for effecting social change" (p. 68) . . . "The theories still to be seen exerting most influence on the model are theories of economic and political democracy and the educational philosophies of Dewey, Kilpatrick and Lindeman, particularly with regard to conceptions of leadership, communal responsibility and forms of group interaction" (p. 69). One of the major limitations of the model, in the view of Papell and Rothman, is the lack of clear differentiation between group work and community organization.

Cohen (1953) and Konopka (1958) acknowledged the influence of Lindeman on their work. Lindeman's interest in and contributions to the development of community organization practice within social work would appear to support the point made by Papell and Rothman.

Konopka, however, moved to a position that distinguishes between the use of groups for individual therapeutic and social action goals (1963).

Klein and others were not willing to countenance a split in group work along the lines suggested by Konopka.

> . . . Klein, Myerson, Rubenstein, and Sirls set forth a reaffirmation of the social action component being indispensable in social groupwork. . . . They contend that there is a unity between social action and individual psychological health and ego strength.
> . . . Grace Coyle strongly believed that the social nature of man grows to its fullest only when he uses himself with and for the benefit of others. . . . Coyle alluded to the importance of social action to the individual actor in addition to the importance of the goal for society or the common good. Although Konopka presents a dichotomy as late as 1963, it seems preferable to postulate that social action is important in ego development and also that work with groups does have a potential for teaching skills in a participatory democracy and for achieving social change. (Klein, 1970 pp. 39-41)

Klein asserts that "we use ourselves, our knowledge and our skills to build democracy in our groups, our agencies, our neighbourhoods and our communities and to develop citizens who know how to live in a democracy" (1953, p. xvi). He sees citizenship education and social action as intertwined. "The members should be helped to understand what can and cannot be done to change conditions, and to learn the techniques for effecting change when the proper occasion arises" (p. 143).

The fact that Klein, Lang (1972), and others needed to reassert the unity of group work practice and to evoke the teachings of Coyle for this purpose, reflects a sense that social action had lost its central position in group work practice and theory and needed to be reclaimed. But this had to take into account new factors that emerged.

The social movements of the 1960's transformed community organization for a decade at least, and inspired many group workers to become more politically active. The concept of "participatory democracy," encouraged by the slogan "maximum feasible participation," had within it the potential to renew interest among group workers in political theory. But this decade was also characterized by anti-intellectualism and anti-professionalism, even within professional ranks, and by a degree of defensiveness on the part of the established services. This was not a climate that tended to incorporate or reincorporate political theory into group work.

The move to systems theory introduced an ecological perspective, holism, and genericism in social work. The effect of this move was to subsume group work (and other methods) under a more abstract formulation, to define society and the polity as "environment," and to transform action into an aspect of transaction. The theoretical elegance of this formulation made it possible to unite social work theory, practice and education under one theoretical umbrella, but failed to take sufficient account of the realities on the ground.

In the extent to which group work writing and teaching reached back to early "democratic" theory, they tended to emphasize aspects of that theory other than the social action role for groups. Group workers continued to insist on their responsibility (and that of all social workers) to engage in social action, and to help group members become better, more responsible citizens, through democratic participation within their groups.

Along the road the concept of the centrality of social action was lost. Even more important, the concept of the centrality of groups in social action and social change processes was lost as well. It is this loss which helps explain the retreat from social action in group work.

THE PLACE OF THE GROUP
IN CONTEMPORARY WRITING

Group workers interested in community oriented practice have sought a bridge between group work and community organization, as others have tried to connect group work and administrative practice (Bakalinsky, 1984, Lewis, 1983, Moore, 1987, Cnaan and Adar, 1987, Imbrogno, 1987, and Gentry, 1987). These have shown how group processes can be used for community work purposes. This emphasis on the group as a tool for achieving community oriented goals, tended to set community organization apart from group work.

The recent work of Hirayama and Hirayama (1986), Pernell (1986), Lee (1986), Wood and Middleman (1989), Lewis (1989), and Breton (1989a, b), using the language of competence, consciousness-raising and empowerment, is suggestive of theory which goes beyond the conceptualizations of the "social goals" model, and its proponents.

Wood and Middleman formulate an approach that is "structural" (1974, 1989). They see their "ideological antecedents" as Mary Richmond, Charlotte Towle, Bertha Reynolds, Harry Lurie, Max Siporin, and Carel Germain rather than the group work pioneers and their associates discussed above. In part, this may be due to the fact that their work is directed at social workers generally rather than group workers.

> The structural approach aims to modify the environment to the needs of the individuals. Social work, theories and practice, has long claimed concern for both persons and environments. But the predominant attention has been focused on the persons, not their situations (perhaps because it seems harder to change situations/environments or because agencies and workers are not paid to do this.
>
> . . . The structural approach asks the practitioner to consider *first* the structural surround before placing the problem(s) within the person of the individual(s) (1989, p. 18).
>
> . . . Social change is not separated from social work, not relegated to specialists within the social work profession (community organizers, planners, social policy-makers). Rather, it is pursued at every level of assignment, every working day by all social workers, and especially by those who must face clients directly. (p. 16)

They refer to "empowerment and advocacy (and social action) groups," using Lee's experience with homeless women. "Working toward empowerment through advocacy entails special strategies and tactics in the political realm, a range of power pressures by the members and worker. Social workers with groups are becoming more knowledgeable in this arena" (p. 207).

The potential strength of the "structural model" is not fully developed in the context of group work. The tendency to see this approach as a way to achieve individual goals and to see the group as means to accomplish this purpose tends to set it apart from group work.

Concepts such as "empowerment" and "advocacy" suggest lines of development towards a more central role for group work and for social action in group work.

Lewis' work with adult groups comes close to defining a more integrated approach to a social role for groups and group work, using ideas derived from liberation theology and feminist theory.

> We are reaching for a philosophical base which will bring greater integration of practice—a more wholistic approach which makes possible both personal development and attention to the development of humane societal conditions within one practice. . . . not as a separate off-shoot more closely identified with community organization, but as an integral part of social group work practice in all of its sites.
>
> . . . It should be apparent that member participants in social work groups are a vital part of the praxis for change, and may have the greatest stake in both defining and working toward that change. The social purpose provides the opportunity for *empowerment*, for active, responsible participation in the social, or public realm (1989).

Lee's practice with the homeless strikes a similar note. Drawing on the ideas of the group work pioneers, as well as the more recent work of Goroff, Tropp, Alissi, Germain, Gitterman, and others, and particularly the interactionist, mutual aid perspective of Schwartz, she blends the personal and the political. She is concerned with helping "the client find in herself the competence to build her self-esteem and relatedness" and to change environments (1987, p. 9).

This requires the development of political skills and perspectives for work with the poor and oppressed. "We need to help people to find the power within themselves, their social networks and communities" (p. 8).

Breton shares the interest of Lewis in liberation theology and the experience of Lee with the homeless. She sees "the political factor" as central for group workers. "We have to question what power we are willing to forego and to what extent we are willing to redefine roles and functions" (1989a, p. 5). In addition, she calls for a critical re-examination of the basic premises underlying the "social action" and "reciprocal" models of practice, if they are to be applied to work with the marginalized and involuntarily disenfranchized. She sees Coyle's educationally oriented approach as tending to focus on individual responsibility and is basically "elitist." She accepts Papell's and Rothman's view that the reciprocal model presupposes "a symbiotic interdependence" between the individual and society; in contrast, oppression presupposes "a breakdown between individual and society" where neither has any expectations of the other (*ibid.*, p. 12).

A "political action model" needs "awareness of the implications of oppression and a political commitment to the oppressed, and leads to defending the interests of the oppressed against those of the oppressors" (*Ibid.*, p. 12).

It is the extra-group, political dimension of conscientization that we are less familiar with or less inclined to digest. This dimension requires that individuals identify not only with a small group in which they feel they belong and in which their direct influence attempts result in a sense of greater personal well-being. The political dimension requires that individuals identify with those people outside the group who share their situation; it requires that they interact with the community of which they and the group are a part, attempting, often indirectly, to influence its institutions in order to bring about social change and greater social justice and well-being. (p. 10)

Breton goes beyond Lee's call for political skills and insists that the model has important implications for the role of the group worker. The model is a power-sharing one. The poor and oppressed must be helped to be "conscientized," "so that they can be the primary agents of their own liberation" (p. 10).

While cognizant of, and committed to the value base at the roots of group work in the settlement, recreation, and progressive education movements, Breton calls for the incorporation of ideas that open the group up to broader social issues and processes and that require a different perspective on the helping process (1989b).

Lewis, Lee, and Breton represent a view of social action that places the group at the center of group work, much as Addams, Coyle and others saw the group as an integral part of the social fabric. Their practice theory has an important political dimension. They recognize that not only the personal is political; practice is also political.

North-American social work has become less ethnocentric. The experience of the poor and the oppressed in the third world has been accompanied by concern for marginal groups within developed society and social work has been opened to the thinking of political theorists like Freire, Guttierez and others in South America, as well as that of Canadians and Europeans. The experience of other countries — Canada, the U.K. and continental Europe — may be quite different, but their analysis may provide useful models for social group work as it seeks to find a path to social action in the contemporary world (Mullender and Ward, 1985).

Continuity for group workers over a century of commitment to social action must integrate groups with their role in society. The role may have shifted from education for democracy to conscientization for liberation.

It also has to do with group workers' roles vis-à-vis their groups and vis-à-vis society — from educator to collaborator in social change.

The thread of continuity must be many-stranded to include political theory as well as theories of human behaviour and social behaviour at the microsocial level. Political theory may have changed — from naive pluralism to a more dynamic sense of the role of conflict and power in society.

But group work needs to continue to recognize that these processes are played out within the group and that they have consequences well beyond the group's boundaries.

Does this require a group work model which separates social action from other purposes and activities in group work? Would such a model be able to incorporate a concern for the needs, rights, goals, and powers of the individual, for achieving a society which is organized to promote these ends, with groups at the center as basic units of social existence and social action? The components of such a model were in place at the beginning. New realities require a new understanding of these same essentials.

BIBLIOGRAPHY

Addams, Jane. *Democracy and Social Ethics*, New York: Macmillan, 1902.
———. *Twenty Years at Hull House with Autobiographical Notes*, New York: Macmillan, 1910.
Bakalinsky, Rosalie. "The Small Group in Community Organization Practice," *Social Work with Groups*, 7(2), 1984, 87-96.
Breton, Margot. "Liberation Theology, Group Work, and the Right of the Poor and Oppressed to Participate in the Life of the Community," *Social Work with Groups*, 1989a, 12(3), 5-18.
———. "Learning from Social Group Work Traditions." Keynote address, 11th Annual Symposium, Association for the Advancement of Social Work with Groups, Montreal, 1989b (mimeo).
Cnaan, R. A. and H. Adar. "An Integrative Model for Group Work in Community Organization Practice," *Social Work with Groups*, 10(3), 1987, 5-24.
Cohen, Nathan C. "E. C. Lindeman—The Teaching and Philosophy," *Proceedings*, National Conference of Social Work, 1953.
Cooley, C. H. *Social Organization: A Study of the Larger Mind*, New York: Scribner, 1909.
Coyle, Grace L. *Social Process in Organized Groups*, New York: Richard R. Smith, 1930.
———. "Group Work and Social Change" (Pugsley Award Lecture), *Proceedings of the National Conference of Social Work*, Chicago: U. of Chicago Press, 1935, 393-405.
———. "The Great Tradition and the New Challenge," *Social Service Review*, 35, 1961, 6-14.
Dewey, John. *The School and Society*. Chicago: U. of Chicago, 1900.
——— and J. H. Tufts. *Ethics*, New York: Holt, 1908.
Follett, Mary Parker. *The New State: Group Organization the Solution of Popular Government*, New York: Longmans, Green, 1920.
Gentry, M. E. "Coalition Formation and Processes," *Social Work with Groups*, 10(3), 1987, 39-54.
Hirayama, H. and K. Hirayama. "Empowerment through Group Participation: Process and Goal," Parnes, M. (Ed.) *Innovations in Social Group Work:*

Feedback from Practice to Theory, New York: The Haworth Press, Inc., 1986, 119-131.

Imbrogno, Salvatore. "Group Work Practices in a Policy System Design," *Social Work with Groups*, 10(3), 1987, 25-37.

Klein, A. F. *Society – Democracy – and the Group*, New York: Association Press, 1953.

———. *Social Work Through Group Process*, Albany: SUNY, 1970.

Konopka, Gisela. *Eduard C. Lindeman and Social Work Philosophy*, Minneapolis: U. of Minnesota Press, 1958.

———. *Social Group Work: a Helping Process*, Englewood Cliffs, N.J.: Prentice-Hall, 1963.

Lang, Norma. "A Broad-Range Model of Practice in Social Group Work," *Social Service Review*, 46(1), 1972, 76-84.

Lee, Judith A. B. "Social Work with Oppressed Populations: Jane Addams Won't You Please Come home?" Lassner, J. et al., *Social Work with Groups: Competence and Values*, New York: The Haworth Press, Inc., 1987, 1-16.

Lee, Judith A. B. and C. R. Swenson. "The Concept of Mutual Aid," Gitterman, A. and L. Shulman (eds.), *Mutual Aid Groups and the Life Cycle*, Itasca, Ill.: Peacock, 1986, 361-380.

Lewis, Elizabeth. "Social Group Work in Community Life: Group Characteristics and Worker Role," *Social Work with Groups*, 1983, 6(2), 3-18.

———. "Social Change and Citizen Action: A Philosophical Exploration for Modern Social Group Work," 11th Annual Symposium, AASWG, Montreal, 1989 (mimeo).

Lindeman, Eduard C. *Social Discovery: An Approach to the Study of Functional Groups*, New York: Republic, 1924.

MacIver, R. M. *The Modern State*, London: Oxford U. Press, 1926.

———. *The Web of Government*, Toronto: Collier Macmillan, 1947.

Middleman, Ruth and Gale Goldberg. *Social Service Delivery: A Structural Approach to Social Work Practice*, New York: Columbia, 1974.

Moore, E. E. "The Group-in-Community as the Unit of Attention in Conceptualizing Social Work with Groups," Lassner, J. et al. (eds), *op. cit.*, 67-79.

Mullender, A. and D. Ward. "Towards an Alternative Model of Social Groupwork," *British Journal of Social Work*, 15, 1985, 155-172.

Papell, C. P. and B. Rothman. "Social Group Work Models: Possession and Heritage," *Journal of Education for Social Work*, 2(2), 1966, 66-77.

Pernell, R. B. "Empowerment and Social Group Work," Parnes, M. (ed.), *op. cit.* 107-117.

Scott, A. F. "Introduction," Addams, Jane, *Democracy and Social Ethics*, Cambridge, Mass.: Harvard U. Press, 1964.

Siporin, Max. "Group Work Method and The Inquiry," Glasser, P. H. and N. S. Mayadas (eds.), *Group Workers at Work: Theory and Practice of the '80's*, Totowa, N.J.: Rowman and Littlefield, 1986, 34-49.

Wood, G. G. and R. R. Middleman. *The Structural Approach to Direct Practice in Social Work*, New York: Columbia, 1989.

Social Change and Citizen Action: A Philosophical Exploration for Modern Social Group Work

Elizabeth Lewis

SUMMARY. This paper explores the import of two selected philosophical/theological perspectives, feminist theory and liberation theology, for social group work practice with citizen groups. Its purposes are to focus on the power of social beliefs and theoretical perspectives to shape the meaning of life circumstances and situations for populations, and either to provide support for group action, or engender resignation or cynical indifference.

Social group work's philosophy of democratic participation and religious commitment to social justice produced a unity of purpose for practitioners. The identification and incorporation of facets of liberation theology and feminist theory offer more current and perhaps sophisticated frames for integrated practice. Both perspectives highlight the centrality of the participant's thinking, knowing and doing both for personal becoming and community renewal.

A profession is identified by the interplay of its belief systems, its values, its purposes, its knowledge bases, and its skill components. In the evolution of social group work practice various of these have enjoyed preeminence. Responsive to the prevailing scientific paradigm, practitioners and theoreticians put great emphasis on knowledge building, and the development of predictive capacity in practice. This paper examines the philosophies which have shaped knowledge acquisition and skill development. It aims to introduce

Elizabeth Lewis, PhD, is Professor, Department of Social Work, Cleveland State University, Euclid Ave. at East 24th Street, Cleveland, OH 44115.

Presented at Eleventh Annual Symposium on Social Work with Groups, Montreal, Quebec, Canada, October 1989.

balance between philosophy and knowledge, and greater congruence between value positions and the philosophy of science, i.e., underlying premises in the pursuit of knowledge.

Two current and developing intellectual/practical arenas are examined for their potential contributions to a more holistic conceptualization of social group work, namely feminist theory and liberation theology. Each has the characteristics of a social movement and has attracted its own adherents and theorists. Each implies a praxis — a set of actions or practices based upon a particular philosophical stance, and thus useful to a practicing profession.

In some ways the development of social group work evolved forward, from beliefs and commitments, and backward, from experiences, to discovery and development of systematic knowledge. Early practice was critiqued as high on affect and commitment but weak on theory, as unscientific in an era of increasing scientific vigor. Later developments may be critiqued for imbalanced attention on "scientific" knowledge bases, methodology or technology — the skill component — without sufficient concern for purpose or mission — the business with which an agent is charged. The inextricable entanglements of philosophy and science, which we identify as theory, further compound the clear articulation of social group work practice. While what follows accents the importance of changed paradigms for knowing, a shift in the philosophy of science, this does not diminish the need for continued pursuit of broader understanding or more skillful practice.

Without extended discussion of philosophical polarities, we note the "idealists" to whom thought is paramount, "materialists" where matter and motion are what counts, and "dualists" where the attempt is to balance "mind and matter." Philosophy differs from theology, dealing with speculation rather than faith. It differs from science because it deals with inquiry rather than "facts" (New Columbia Encycl. p. 2, 133).

American social work, group work included, has ranged widely in the pursuit of knowledge bases for practice. This has been based on a U.S. philosophy of science, particularly pragmatism and logical positivism, where meaning is derived from empirical observation. For the past several decades the logical positivist approach has dominated our search for knowledge and meaning. However, since at least the early '70's this heavy emphasis on the empirical has been challenged by social work researchers and theorists as well as practitioners. It is interesting to note that women have posed many of the critiques as well as alternative paradigms.

Polar positions in the philosophy of science pose particular hardships on the development of social group work. Small groups, in social work and out, are the bridging structures between persons and larger social entities. They have a duality in sometimes being ends in themselves, and sometimes means to other, more external, ends. Theoretically polar positions force practitioners to make choices between these purposes.

Social group work was a North American invention. It had multiple roots in education, in religion, in recreation. Each of these disciplines had its own purposes. Initially, the development of group members, intellectually, spiritually, and physically was interwoven with more social purposes, the socializing of ethnic, immigrant populations to the liberal tradition of democratic participation.

The historic era of the '20's was reformist and pragmatic. The major philosophic bases were derived from John Dewey. Experience was the basis for learning. Social group work was identified as a social movement, springing from the organizations whose purposes were *societal*, and whose concerns were for *populations*. This early practice was praised for its philosophical commitments but critiqued for its lack of a "scientific base."

An examination of settlements as host agencies for group practice may recall the qualitative nature of their inquiry. The live experience of neighbors, usually shared by the "residents" of the house, guided the understanding of life conditions and causes. Thus, interventions could be aligned to desired outcomes. The cooperation of settlement workers with sociologists and their field research, particularly in Chicago, served to strengthen a qualitative methodology.

The move from a wide practice incorporating several disciplines to closer identification with social work led to greater reliance on personality theory and attention to within-group phenomena. The capacity to manipulate the within-group variables in an empirical pursuit of scientific practice led to an emphasis on methodology, of technologies for within-group change.

The group itself as a social entity became a prime object of study.

Internal group processes, perhaps because they are accessible to scientific manipulation and measurement, gave practice a degree of scientific credence. It certainly appears more difficult to chart the impact and effectiveness of specific group interactions on the social fabric, however proximate the target.

The era of model building, with all of its richness and diversity, can be identified by its conflicting philosophical views of the nature of humans in society, and the overriding acceptance of individualism. The shift from movement to method, the close identification with social work (case work) through joining the NASW and the transfer of responsibility for a social focus from worker with group to the professional organization all resulted in present practice emphasis.

Papell and Rothman (1966) in their famous "Models" paper identified the problems for practitioners and theorists in determining the societal functions for social group work. Should it be provision and prevention (the earliest thrust), restoration and rehabilitation, or some combination of both? An underlying argument is whether the person determines the state of the society or whether the society determines the state of the person. This reflects the philosophically polar positions of mind or matter. The "social goals" model is built upon the belief that the person can impact society through a sense of "social consciousness" and "responsibility" for "community."

The remedial model builds on the restorative, rehabilitative function, a focus on person. Ultimately, the clinical cast of much current social group work practice is supported by agency purposes which are therapeutic and rehabilitative and is based on a strong deterministic philosophy. It lends itself to empirical research and thus claims scientific validity in the empirical mode.

The reciprocal model represents a dual stance. The *group* is the central focus of attention. Schwartz, the prime initiator of the model, identified relationships as key and worker responsibilities as aiding members to sort out with him/her meanings, obstacles, requirements and actions in no pre-determined mode. In 1966 none of the models were fully developed. Yet each was based on a philosophy of science which sought to explain the nature of human reality.

CRITIQUES OF LOGICAL POSITIVISM/DETERMINISM

In the last decade, an impressive array of critiques of logical positivism by social work researchers and scholars emerged. These were seen as a problem of fit between method of inquiry and value bases. A full inventory is beyond the scope of this paper. None focus specifically on the impact on social group work but have useful insights in the search for an integrating practice. Zimmerman (*SSR* 1989) identifies the problems of *determinism* in the polar philosophical positions — i.e., ideational or material determinants. He notes continuing problems for researchers and practitioners of *unpredictability* and *equifinality* in understanding human action. [See Heineman (1981), Scott (1989), Wagner (1989), Piele (1988), Whyte (1984), Witkin and Gottschalk (1988), Weick (1983, 1987), Rodwell (1987), Dean and Fenby (1989), Goldstein (1986).] Some of the ideas expressed as alternatives to empiricism include: An explicitly critical theory (Habermas), humans as active agents, theory that accounts for the life experience of clients, attention to language, theory that makes sense cognitively, morally and politically (Witkin and Gottschalk); Liberation, the maximization of each person's and group's ability to act and give shape to their own destiny and promote social justice, (Weick); Existentialism, critical theory, deconstruction (Dean and Fenby); Naturalistic approaches which meet the explanatory needs of the profession without relying on either ideational or material determinants (Zimmerman); Focus on the nature of reality, the relationship of knower to known, the impossibility of generalization, the impossibility of causal linkages, the role of values in inquiry (Rodwell); Inquiry in the natural setting, the essential position of the human instrument, the utilization of tacit knowledge, qualitative methods, negotiated outcomes, ideographic interpretations, tentativeness, (Rodwell).

Most of these alternatives in the philosophy of science seek to maintain discipline and rigor in method of inquiry without the limitation of a predetermined first cause. These are useful developments for advancing social group work practice. We are reaching for a philosophical base which can integrate practice — a holistic approach to bring both personal development and attention to the creation of humane societal conditions within one practice.

The need for a philosophical base to integrate social purpose into all of social group work, not as a separate off-shoot more closely identified with community organization, is apparent in the continued vulnerability of women, of minorities of color, of poor persons, of single parent families, of displaced workers, among the many populations served by social workers. These vulnerabilities stem from socially defined statuses which are institutionalized in the structures of society. They are maintained by attitudes, behaviors and the language of definition.

THE IDENTIFICATION OF SOCIAL PURPOSE

What is meant by social purpose integral to social group work practice? While social change is often presaged by individual advocates, writers and speakers, the process requires collective action. The action may take on the dimensions of a social movement, wherein diverse populations and small groups converge in the identification of a situation generally accepted as normal, as practically disadvantaging to them. It is redefined in its troublesome aspects, "deconstructed." This new definition helps sensitize others to their own disadvantagement or vulnerability. The deconstruction of the occurrence or idea, the identification of its components, and how it disadvantages some while advantaging others has been identified as "conscientization" (Paolo Freire), consciousness raising, in the women's movement, or as the Chinese say, "speaking bitter." While this process may be cathartic to its participants, social change requires the development of possible courses of action, selection of one or several, taking action, and evaluating outcomes. It further requires the *active* engagement of members of the vulnerable population, as well as "helpers," professionals, religious, and educators, in this exploration and action. It necessitates a critical mass of adherents working toward a reconstruction of the social fabric, a praxis for change. Member participants in social work groups are a vital part of the praxis for change, and may have the greatest stake in defining and working toward that change. The social purpose provides the opportunity for *empowerment*, for active, responsible participation in the social or public realm.

Why select feminist theory and liberation theology for analysis, and for their potential for reintroducing social purpose into social group work? Each provides illustrative material relevant to the goal of holistic practice. Both are social movements with characteristics similar to early social group work. Unlike early practice, there is in each a strong explication of the method of inquiry (the philosophy of science) or an attempt to operationalize the spiritual or value component. By itself each lacks some components (feminist theory perhaps less so). Together they present female and male world views. Together they cover both ideational and material/historical facets of the human condition.

FEMINIST THEORY

Feminist theory examines the conditions of life, beliefs about, and status of women in society. Women make up at least half the population of North American society and are clearly vulnerable by many measures: economic, social, political, spiritual. They are the major recipients of public welfare and mental health services. Female-headed families increasingly are the poor and the homeless. Women also are the major deliverers of social services. Feminist theory has had an impact on the public consciousness of women's vulnerabilities, on some social policies, and on family structure. It has shaped both women's and men's consciousness of self and of "appropriate" relations between the sexes. Exploration of its utility for an increased social component in social group work practice seems useful.

Feminist theory is not unitary in its orientations. It has been classified as liberal, radical or Marxist. Proponents of these positions project a world of equality with men, a world of dominance by women/needing no men, or a world of economic control by women, (where economics is the major determinant of power). Given these differing positions, what seem to be major contributions of feminist theory? These are first in methodology: The reclaiming of her–story, i.e., the search for and inclusion of women's contributions to social history. The identification of women's leadership in the public arena, (albeit circumscribed by the idea that women's place is in the home), a methodology which ascribes meaning and importance to women's experience–the power of women to identify and define their own importance as women, to validate their identity, separate from the definitions of men. The exploration and critiquing of language, as conveyor of ideas and thus a major influence of actions. The critical analysis of organizations and institutions which systematically limit women's opportunities and reinforce a second class status on them.

Feminist theory recognizes the validity of what is called tacit knowledge, the validity of affect, or felt meaning, what group workers have called "practice wisdom," the inability to abstract the knower, i.e., the worker, from the known, the members, the importance of the natural setting, i.e., the lived experience, in this case the members' experience within the group, and the members' collective experiences of the wider contexts of life, i.e., how they see and interpret their experiences beyond the group. The personal is political. The idea of negotiated outcomes seems to be part and parcel of good social group work practice, i.e., what the members and worker can come to through the conjoint interactions and exchanges in the group. Feminist theory pursues a non-linear process of understanding which suggests a more tentative stance, non-generalizable, and non-deterministic. This should feel familiar to group workers. Feminist theory requires an active, participatory stance among the participants, in definitions, understandings, goal setting, defining objectives, actions, and evaluation. Applied to social group work, this means negotiated contributions, not worker or agency dominance but mutual agreement, not passivity but contributions according to talents and rights.

The major contribution of feminist theory to a more social praxis with groups is in a methodology which is specifically egalitarian, participatory, and validating of each member's life experience in context.

LIBERATION THEOLOGY

Liberation theology, focused on the poor and the vulnerable, is "a systematic, disciplined reflection on Christian faith and its implications" Berryman (1987). Liberation theology has its parallels in the "social gospel," in trying to move from strictly theological to practical applications. It goes farther in that it is a *critique* of

economic structures. "Peoples poverty is largely a product of the way society is structured."
It is:

1. "An interpretation of Christian faith out of suffering, struggle, and hope;
2. A critique of society and the ideologies sustaining it;
3. A critique of the activity of the church from the perspective of the poor (Berryman, 1987)."

It has parallels with feminism and Black theology. It is a manifestation of a world-wide movement for human emancipation. It has a major emphasis on "praxis" — practicality (Berryman, 1987). While liberation theology is largely a South America development, its importance has spread to other predominantly Catholic countries, and to parts of Africa. Some of its themes parallel feminist theory and social group work as a movement: As a process of inculturation, in Africa — in reclaiming African culture and beliefs, the reclaiming of indigenous culture within the church, "getting the missionaries off their backs," assisting persons to be the artisans of their own destiny; looking at history to retrieve the past; A manifestation of economic democracy, or as Reuther (1989) identifies, democratic socialism; A way of economic restructuring by the development of small, "base" communities, limited areas within the larger society. Berryman (1987) and McKnight (*Social Policy* 1987) identify a parallel move for urban communities to become economically productive for their own needs rather than importing all resources from outside.

Liberation theology has been critiqued by feminists as primarily a male enterprise. Its major proponents have been Catholic clergymen, members of a historically paternalistic institution. The church has been unwilling to deal with a critique of paternalism. In the development of liberation theology men have been expected to deal with the public, economic aspects, women with the "pastoral work." Catholic feminist theology has been much more radical than liberation theology in its critique of Christianity. Daly (1973) seems willing even to repudiate Christianity itself, if this will free women from domination by the church.

The church has critiqued liberation theology because it appeared to be based on a belief in material determinism. Its proponents have defended its emphasis on the economic structures of society and their impact on the poor and tried to apply theological principles in changing the material conditions of the poor. Some examples of a determinist stance: "A person's social behaviors to a large extent is a product of existing social structures and his/her position in those structures and not a product of his own impartial thought; behavior is changed through change in structures, and structures are changed as much or more by pressure than by reason. In advanced social structures, the degree of liberation is in direct proportion to the participation of the masses in creating them," Ramos (1988) p. 59. "Liberation theology requires an attitude toward political authority that is both critical and responsible. It is a call to a constant struggle to establish justice and defend the life of the mind and the spirit." These last two quotes would seem to be in opposition to a materialist philosophy, perhaps indicative of an attempt to bridge the mind-matter dichotomy.

The major contribution of liberation theology is its insistence on participation in the economic and political spheres of life by the persons most vulnerable to its injustices. It is a substantive contribution to practice, added to the methodological contributions of feminist theory.

We have been attempting to identify philosophical developments which will support a group work practice that enables members to critique, deconstruct, and reconstruct the structures and experiences of life for the membership. The group experience provides the medium to reshape consciousness and the arena for changed ways of thinking, acting, and speaking, to achieve the confidence and competence to reshape everyday experiences and structures of life. The group is not only the medium, but also becomes the instrument through which members can develop that sense of community and mutual support which is needed in the process of social change.

Social group workers who derived their values from a Judeo-Christian tradition calling for respect for persons, self-determination, fairness, equity and democratic participation, may be conflicted when they discover these values in more or less authoritarian, paternalistic institutions. We have separated the domains of church and state, or what might be construed the private and public worlds, or, pushing a bit, the spiritual and material facets of life. A philosophical perspective, and process of scientific inquiry to bridge these parallel and intertwined perspectives is needed. Feminist theory and liberation theology offer some guides for this integration and the stimulus to reintroduce the social purposes into group work practice.

REFERENCES

Berryman, Phillip, *Liberation Theology*, Pantheon Books, NY, 1987.

Cove, James, H., "Martin Luther King, Jr., and the Third World," Chapter 3, in Ellis and Maduro, *The Future of Liberation Theology: Essays in Honor of Gustavo Guttierez.*

Daly, Mary, *Beyond God the Father*, Beacon Press, Boston, 1973.

Dean, Ruth G., and Fenby, Barbara, "Exploring Epistemologies: Social Work Action as a Reflection of Philosophical Assumptions," *Journal of Social Work Education*, 25 (1), Winter 1989, 46-54.

Ellis, Marc and Maduro, Otto, *The Future of Liberation Theology: Essays in Honor of Gustavo*, Orbis Books, Maryknoll, NY, 1989.

Freire, Paolo, *Pedagogy of the Oppressed*, Continuum, NY, 1990 (repub.).

Goldstein, Howard, "Toward the Integration of Theory and Practice: A Humanistic Approach, *Social Work*, 31 (1986) 352-357.

Heineman, Martha, (Peiper), "The Obsolete Scientific Imperative in Social Work Research," *Social Service Review*, 55 (3) 264-284, September 1981.

McKnight, John L., "Regenerating Community," *Social Policy*, Winter 1987, 54-58.

Papell, Catherine P., and Rothman, Beulah, "Social Group Work Models: Possession and Heritage," *Journal of Education for Social Work*, 2 (Fall 1966), 66-77.

Peiper, Martha Heineman, "Critique, Comments on Peile," *Social Service Review*, 562 (3) September 1988, 535-536.

Peile, Colin, "Research Paradigms in Social Work: From Stalemate to Creative Synthesis," *Social Service Review*, 62 (1) March 1988, 1-19.

Ramos, Joseph, Chapter 3, "Reflection on *Gustavo* Theology of Liberation" (50-60) p. 59.

Reuther, Rosemary, "Religion and Society: Sacred Canopy vs. Prophetic Critique," Chapter 23 in *Ellis* and *Maduro, The Future of Liberation Theology*, 172-176.

Rodwell, Mary K., "Naturalistic Inquiry: An Alternative Model for Social Work Assessment," *Social Service Review*, 61 (2) 231-246.

Scott, Dorothy, "Meaning Construction and Social Work Practice," *Social Service Review*, 63 (1), 39-51.

Wagner, David, "Radical Movements in the Social Services: A Theoretical Framework," *Social Service Review*, 63 (2) 264-284.

Weick, Ann, "Reconceptualizing the Philosophical Perspectives of Social Work," *Social Service Review*, 61 (2) 218-230.

Witkin, Shirley L., Gottschalk, Shimon, "Alternative Criteria for Theory Evaluation," *Social Service Review* 62, (2) June 1988, 211-224.

Zimmerman, Jerome H., "Determinism, Science and Social Work," *Social Service Review*, 63 (1) March 1989, 52-63.

New Columbia Encyclopedia, p. 2, 133.

ADDED READINGS

Alissi, Albert, "Social Group Commitments and Perspectives," Chapter 1, 5-35 in Alissi, Albert, ed., *Perspectives on Social Group Work,* Free Press, NY, 1980.

Anderson, Gerald H., ed., and Stransky, Thomas C.S.P., Mission Trends #4, *Liberation Theologies in North America and Europe*, Paulist Press, NY, 1979.

Boff, Leonardo and Boff, Clovis, *Liberation Theology*, Harper & Row, San Francisco, 1986. (trans Portuguese) paper.

Guiterrez, Gustavo, "Theology of Liberation" in Novak, Michael, ed., *Liberation South, Liberation North*, 59-92.

Marins, Jose, and Team, *Basic Ecclesiastical Communities*, Claritian Publications, Quezon, Philippines, 1983, (paper).

Novak, Michael, ed., *Liberation Theology and the Liberal Society*, American Enterprise Institute, Washington, D.C., 1987.

———, *Liberation South, Liberation North*, American Enterprise Institute, Washington, D.C., 1981.

Middleman, Ruth and Goldberg Gale, "Toward the Quality of Social Group Work Practice," in Leiderman, Marcos et al., eds., *Roots and New Frontiers*, The Haworth Press, Inc., NY, 1988.

Sigmond, Paul E., "Liberation Theology: An Historical Evaluation," monograph, The Wilson Center, 1986.

Wilson, Gertrude, "From Theory to Practice: A Personalized History," in Roberts, W., and Northen, Helen, *Theories of Social Work with Groups*, Columbia University Press, 1976.

Social Action, Empowerment and Social Work — An Integrative Theoretical Framework for Social Work and Social Work with Groups

Silvia Staub-Bernasconi

SUMMARY. This article outlines a theoretical framework for social work, social groupwork, and social action based on an evolutionary general systems theory as a *challenge to the dominating Parsonian functionalist perspective*. Its main focus is on the inner, symbolic barriers to effective social action which can be eliminated by a sound theoretical base. The systemic view requires (a) *multi-level-diagnosis* of social problems as a means of relating private troubles to public political issues, (b) conceptualization of *specific problem-dimensions* as object-base (Gegenstand) for social work theory, and (c) development of *problem-centered action lines*, especially methods of empowerment and changing power-structures accessible to social work. The proposed framework may facilitate an international approach to building theories of social work in relation to societal structure and power.

1. SOCIAL MOVEMENTS AND PROFESSIONAL SOCIAL ACTION

In a comparison of political with professional social action, *political social action*, such as the trade union, civil rights, feminist, ecological and peace movements, can be seen as responses to soci-

Silvia Staub-Bernasconi, PhD, Dipl. Social Worker/Sociologist is Professor of social work, social action and social philosophy at the School of Social Work Zurich, University of Trier/BRD and Freiburg/CH. Her address is School of Social Work, Zurich, Bederstr. 115, CH-8002 Zurich, Switzerland.

etal tensions due to illegitimate power. They mostly deal with *one single or dominant issue* (justice, participation, peace, abortion, political voting, pollution, etc.). Research shows, that movements with one single issue and a strong organizational structure are most efficient in reaching their goals (Gamson, 1975).

Social action in social work is seen here as a professional effort to bring into public discourse issues which, according to the consensus between power-holders and the public, should remain in the shadow of public debate, but *also in the shadow of the great social movements*. All great movements have members and leaders from different educational and economic backgrounds and, thus, many human and social resources from which they can benefit. Social work is professionally bound to work on *cumulative problem situations and issues* such as poverty and its multiple psychic, social and cultural consequences, deprivation and oppression, violence, etc. It has to do with scarce resources and structural as well as ideological barriers erected by power-holders and service agencies. Current efficiency norms won't work here (Piven & Cloward, 1977). Escape into medical-therapeutic models of practice — even of private practice focused on individual change — has become a problem-solution of professionals for inherent structural difficulties. Others are suffering burnout symptoms which are not signals of over-work, but expressions of an enormous asymmetry between responsibilities for society-based problems without equivalent rights and power. This paper tries to suggest, in outline form, how to remove some inner limits of practice and education for social (group) work.

2. THE PRIVATE IS POLITICAL — THE POLITICAL IS PRIVATE: MULTILEVEL LOCAL AND GLOBAL THINKING

According to many past and current ideologies and (economic, psychological, socio-psychological) theories, society doesn't really exist! What exists is the individual — subject to the laws of privacy, personal freedom, private enterprise and property. According to a new debate, even organizations are treated as individuals (Dan-Cohen, 1986). Social problems are thus private problems to be solved privately.

Professional and systemic thinking about social problems requires a perception of societal reality at different levels of social organization—individuals, small and large (extended) families, small and large groups (along ethnic, religious, gender and racial lines), small and large territorial communities (from neighborhoods to urban centers, regions, nations and world society), and finally, small and large (transnational) organizations. The awareness by individuals of their social memberships in all these social systems is generally low. But there is even less awareness of the complex causalities and interaction effects of these multiple social systems on the individual and vice versa. This explains why, not only politicians, but most people are "social analphabets." To avoid this danger, professional thinking requires a theoretical framework going beyond reflections on interaction between "individual and environment"; it has to deal with levels of organization, structures and processes—encompassing physical, biological, psychic, social and cultural reality and the evolutionary as well as causal links between them (Laszlo, 1987; Bunge, 1974ff; Staub-Bernasconi, 1983, 1986, 1988a, 1989).

A social group is a level of social organization with its own problems, a level possibly causing problems for other levels or an instrument for problem solving on its own or another level. *Social work with groups* would then have at least three meanings: (a) work within the group, because it is the richest resource system for problem solving and help for its members; (b) work with a group, whose structure and processes are the main subjective or objective problem area, and (c) work with groups as an instrument to reach goals outside the group, in another social subsystem. The three approaches can be combined. But before the worker can decide on the work to be done, he/she has to solve the task of multilevel problem definition.

Consider the problem of a youngster with a pattern of high school truancy attracted to a streetgang as defined by a worrying mother:

- On the *individual* level it may be a problem of undetected legastheny, causing anxiety about exams and grades, to which the youngster's solution is escape. The risk of school dropout and unemployment are the next predictable problems on the individual level. Diagnostic projection and knowledge might visualize homelessness, drugs and criminality as possible developments.

- School anxieties and truancy may also be influenced by *family* constellations. It could be passive resistance, because there is no possibility of conflict articulation and problem solving within the family due to paradoxical family communication or the effect of housing and poor income. Not being fixed on family problem diagnosis, one would ask further questions,
- about the *neighborhood* — racial or ethnic conflicts impinging on *gang*-formation, opportunities for leisure activities, alternative rewarding social memberships, which are possibly in sharp contrast to the rewards of
- the school as *educational organization and the class as group*. The hidden curriculum might have a built-in-program of negative self-fulfilling phrophecies in regard to members of ethnic, racial, religious or sexual minorities. This can lead to the question of
- the problems of the *professional group* of teachers, their own education, the curriculum demands or feelings of helplessness to deal with prejudices and violence in the classroom within a deteriorating neighborhood.
- The diagnostic track of housing and neighborhood conditions would raise questions about *organizations* — political parties, ownership or landlord organizations — which block building rehabilitation, innovation and state investment for housing. Today, an expanding global economy would require diagnosis on
- the *world level*. A global real estate market seeks property in urban centers all over the world at any price for the establishment of headquarters and "Regional Profit Centers" as bases of operation for *stateless trans-national organizations*.

Given this social problem-picture, who is the client to be served or changed? This is a matter of definition, based on information and causal attribution. It becomes a professional definition by the following criteria: Who suffers? In what way is this suffering directly or indirectly causally linked with other social levels because of open or hidden memberships and influences? What knowledge do we have about this? Consider school dropout. Is it really a legastheny and thus a problem on the neurobiological level which requires "nothing but" careful handling by the teacher or perhaps a self-help group of pupils? If not, how are school dropout-problems connected with housing problems, the professional status and possible resignation of teachers, the school-organization within a poor neighborhood and/or the global real estate market? Even if the intervention level is clear—is "social action" or "empowerment" the most appropriate direction for work?

The very difference between political and professional thinking and action is, that the former tries to reduce complexity, sometimes in a demagogic way, and that the latter has to make things more complicated. It could be the base for a diagnostic dialogue between representatives of the traditional professional territories of case, group, community and planning-administration work and lead to concerted action. Isn't it the unique, fascinating and challenging feature of social work, that its diagnostic tools and intervention strategies encompass all levels of social organization?

3. EMPOWERMENT IS THE ANSWER – TELL ME FIRST WHAT IS THE PROBLEM?

Social work has a tradition of level-specific methods of work with individuals, families, and groups, life-space and streetwork, community and organizational work. For a long time specialization has followed these lines, although historically, the theoretical and practical pioneers (Jane Addams, Florence Kelley, Bertha Reynolds, Mary Richmond, Alice Salomon, etc.) integrated all these approaches within their own person, thinking and doing (Staub-Bernasconi, 1986, 1989). Ongoing differentiation and specialization within society and the profession generated both a search for a generic approach to social work as well as further differentiation in regard to special client groups (women, homeless, new immigrants, physically handicapped, mentally ill). Neither solution has answered satisfactorily the crucial question for action theory development in social work: *"What is the problem base of social work?"* Notions of *"people coping with environmental demands"* (Bartlett, 1970, p. 99), and thus social dysfunction, are vague and do not deal with power issues. Even in an elaborated functional framework (Germain & Giterman, 1980; Chess & Norlin, 1988), the theoretical notion of power is lacking. Functionalism still dominates the discussion (McIntire, 1986; Staub-Bernasconi, 1983, 1986). This black hole concerning the object and problem-base (Gegenstand) of social work is one reason why, especially in the German area, social work theory is in stagnation (Staub-Bernasconi, 1988). It is not so much the level of social intervention, or the function or goal (therapeutic/remedial, preventive, reciprocal or social goal achievement), but the *problem-reality and its dimensions* which should guide the choice of methods in social work (Staub-Bernasconi, 1986, 1988b).

This also applies to the discussion of empowerment and social action. If empowerment is the answer, one would have to ask, for what problem? Empowerment can't be the remedy for all problems of social work, but it can help promote discussion about power in general, legitimate and illegitimate power structures, and methods to approach some basic problem configurations. They all have to do with the production of and accessibility to scarce goods — money, work, knowledge, housing, property, land, infrastructure, etc. In a survey about power notions in social work, McIntire (1986) summarizes:

> With few exceptions, the literature that reports on social (development) work makes no specific connections with existing theories of power. (p. 12)
> The views of Parsons and the functionalists have been extremely influential in Western (American) social work and social welfare thought, in casework, groupwork, organizational development and in the form of the social service system . . . Certainly his views on poverty and deviance shaped the nature of social services and agencies for three decades. One might hazard the view that this influence has contributed to the absence of explicit examination of the dynamics of power in dyadic relationships, families and groups. (p. 28)

Parsons' "Four-problem paradigm" and concept of power assumes consensus or competition over values, but precludes conflict over distribution of goods, contradictions between social groups or classes and the social construction of illegitimate dominance. Being forced to look for dysfunctional role fulfillment of individuals in regard to societal functions precludes the question of how functional a society, its economic and political system and its social agencies are for the individual (see my analysis of Germain & Giterman's "functionalism": Staub-Bernasconi 1986, pp. 43-44).

What follows is a brief conceptual outline of the *problem-base of social work*, of which power-problems are an important part:

(1) Individual, familial and organizational resource problems (multiple dimensions of poverty): For the individual, they include poor physical health, disablement, and impaired attractivity — *problems of the body*. In addition we have pollution, congestion and poor environment — summarized as *socio-ecological problems* in the dwelling or workplace. Resource or *socio-economic problems* are lack of education, work, income, housing, medical care, social insurances, and also lack of medical or socio-cultural infrastructure. What follows, if we consider individuals and social units as information-processing organisms, are *problems of information processing* or epistemology — emotional problems as well as problems of normative evaluation and cognition. The products of information processing are images, codes, values, plans, etc. The *problems of symbolization and modelling* the world and the people in it can be inadequate images, code deficiencies, low self-esteem, unattainable lifegoals and therefore alienation, social prejudices, human-despising values.

The next problem dimensions refer to *behavioral functioning (individuals)* and problems of *social role construction and the division of labor (families, organizations)*. Thus, the often used term "coping problems" can mean lack of competencies or creativity, social deviance or social disorganization and anomie. Social memberships — ascribed and self-chosen — are resources. Their lack we call *social isolation*.

(2) Problems of asymmetrical exchange relationships: Within horizontal social interactions with peers or in labor, knowledge and other markets, the above personal or organizational *resources become "exchange-media"*: Poor and low quality resources make for an *unattractive exchange-partner* and the likelihood of asymmetri-

cal interaction without chances for equalization, and thus, further decline of resources and increased risks of social isolation.

(3) Problems of powerlessness and the power-structure: Within horizontal as well as vertical social interactions (i.e., the interaction between partners with equal and unequal resources), the personal and collective resources/exchange media become "power sources." These form the base for the building and consolidation of power-structures.

Powerlessness is a result of relationships in which poor resources lead to low social attractiveness and thus to very low chances to control one's own life by the access to the resources of others. The more and qualitatively different resources one has, the better one can control other resources, people, and ideas according to the individual's and organization's goals and long-term interests.

Within this framework social power structures and social sub-systems are seen as socially problematic or unjust, when and only when they don't meet basic human needs and inhibit the fulfillment of legitimate aspirations, although they may be very functional for power-holding societal groups and the integration of society (Staub-Bernasconi 1983, Bunge 1989). An aspiration is legitimate, if it can be fulfilled by individual or cooperative achievements without hindering the meeting of basic needs of other members. To quote a system philosopher (Bunge, 1989):

> A society has a just social structure if every member of the society can attain well-being, or even reasonable happiness, without others suffering from it. Otherwise the social structure is unjust. (pp. 50, 372) . . . A society is externally just if and only if it does not hinder the development of other societies. A society is just if and only if it is both internally and externally just. (p. 373)

Thus, we distinguish between *"inhibiting or hindering power-structures"* and *"constraining power-structures,"* assuming that reality is some sort of a mixture. Totalitarian and authoritarian societies are almost entirely socially and functionally integrated, but unjust societies. Constraining power-structures are constructed by distribution and behavioral norms which adapt scarce resources, goods, man/womanpower and ideas to human needs and legitimate aspirations. A society doesn't have to be rich, to be just.

It is possible to discern *four different problem dimensions of inhibiting power-structures*. The *first* refers to the distribution of goods and resources to individuals, families, organizations and nations. The *second* considers the social organization of men and women for the purpose of labor and social control (division of labor; decision- and sanctioning-power). The *third* relates to the dominant symbols, ideas or ideology for the legitimation of power-arrangements and the *fourth* concerns the problem of influence, coercion and violence.

Problems of "inhibiting power" exist:

- when "the few" deprive "the many" of control over (scarce) resources so that the gains go to the few and the costs and losses go to the many. These are *problems of social distribution and stratification* exemplified in feudal caste structures, classic capitalist class structure, neo-feudalism, racism, ethnocentrism and sexism, etc.;
- when the division of labor stabilizes exploitative hierarchical relationships: *problems of domination*
- resulting in physical abuse, economic exploitation, cultural colonialization, psychic or technocratic manipulation inherent in the social construction of social systems;
- when these social arrangements are legitimized by constitution and supported by law and social norms, which refer to god, nature, history or even culture as immutable, everlasting "ideas": *problems of legitimation* of discriminatory stratification and illegitimate dominance;
- when *force and violence* are used to reinforce and stabilize these forms of inhibiting power structures.

(4) Problems of non-existing or arbitrary social criteria or values: Human and social conditions are evaluated based on universal or particular and local values, i.e., values underlying "The Declaration of Human Rights," "The Declaration of Social Rights" or national laws, etc. Problematic is the lack of such values, i.e., in gene- and bio-technology, in global business and research prac-

tices. Problematic is also the arbitrary use of existing values and resulting norms in court, in university, and business regarding the allocation of resources, career promotion for minority-members, and in social work, regarding the assignment of subsidies, housing and work for deserving or not-deserving clients.

Problem-Centered Social Action in Social Work

Based on this frame of reference, these problem dimensions serve as the basis for selection of theory guided "methods of social action." They also suggest, how education in methods and skills of social work in the broad sense could be reconceptualized.

(1) Resource-Mobilization: This action line responds to the most pressing, existential needs of human beings lacking resources for physical, psychic and social survival in a depriving environment. It is actually the oldest "method" of social work and was relevant on all social levels, starting with the systematic sociodemographic analysis of depressed areas and the socio-economic situation of immigrants, women, the unemployed. Hull House, the Chicago settlement, is a good example of the use of groups for problem-level solutions, but also as a means to intervene on other, more complex social levels for resource-mobilization purposes, i.e., better sanitary, work, loan, housing and educational conditions. *Streetwork* is a form of resource-mobilization of first help on the street, a social territory or life-space level. Newer differentiations and specializations in this action field are *"grassroot-work"* as resource-mobilization from below, *"social planning"* as resource-mobilization from above and *"social management"* as internal and external resource allocation by social agencies.

(2) Consciousness development: Groups are the arena for consciousness raising about one's own and others' problem situations. Many techniques which are directed to emotional catharsis, establishing norms and cognitive insights (i.e., Konopka, 1983) can also be used for raising insight about societal processes and structures. The suggestion here is to complete these techniques, which stem from psychoanalysis and humanistic psychology with techniques stemming from work with severely deprived, even illiterate, people such as the methods of Paolo Freire (1980) relying heavily on im-

ages/pictures, linguistic analysis and the concentration on "generative concepts" and "themes" of the poor and oppressed.

(3) Symbolic or cultural change and innovation: The point of departure here is the deficiency of cognitive maps, hindering images of self and others, prejudices, feelings of meaninglessness, lack of life-goals: On the group level several techniques for better information processing, to change prejudices or to find new life-goals are familiar. They analyze and reconstruct the biography and the social context (i.e., Schwartz, 1976) and try to develop future scenarios.

(4) Social or coping skills training: Much groupwork has been an answer for behavioral problems, especially destructive behavior (Vinter, 1967); but there is also a long tradition of learning new social skills, experience democracy and leadership within groups (Wilson & Ryland, 1949), later enriched by methods of psycho- and sociodrama.

(5) Social networking – Mediating: This is a response to psychic and social isolation, especially to the breakdown of neighborhood relations in urban centers. It also attempts to develop mediation techniques in regard to paradoxical communication and asymmetrical exchange of resources in general (Schwartz, 1976).

(6) Empowerment as work with power-sources and power-structures: American social workers have never seen themselves as social revolutionaries and European workers do not – except in the 1960s – see themselves engaged in great societal transformation. Yet, to concentrate on societal power overlooks the power in dyadic (i.e., male-female), family and group-relationships, or in the work place, the social agency or the neighborhood. Fixation on "grand theory" and "grand changes" obscures the fact, that change can take place within easily accessible structures as pioneering social laboratories (Addams, 1930; Alinsky 1971).

Social workers often forget that, at their beginning, women social workers organized internationally against war, hunger, child abuse, disease at home and abroad, using action groups and social organizations as their main vehicles (Grosser, 1973). Although publicly ridiculed, they visited political leaders, built lobbies, and suggested "peaceful methods" and new "social contracts" to resolve national and international conflicts. At a new phase of transition to global society it is time to revitalize this tradition.

(7) Methods of public, official and unofficial discourse about values: We look for guidelines and skills for public discussion of ethical dilemmas (i.e., abortion) and handling media based on sound knowledge and fair argument.

The combination of specific intervention levels and their actors with problem-based methods can be called *concerted-action*. *Empowerment as an action line* has, within this theoretical framework, a precise social indication: problems of power as lack of access to goods/resources, domination, illegitimacy of power structures and violence.

4. DEVELOPING PRACTICE KNOWLEDGE FOR THE EMPOWERMENT OF CLIENTS AND SOCIAL WORK AS A PROFESSION

It is the problem which determines the required knowledge and skills and not the other way round. This applies especially to European adaptation of methods developed outside social work. It also applies to social work educational curricula set up by American experts in the Third World. It is the Third World which sees most clearly the "power blindness" of American social work—due to functionalism in all its facets (Schulze, 1983).

Starting with problem-definition on different social levels has the great advantage of facilitating the integration of badly needed basic knowledge outside social work literature, including the contributions of Weber, Marx, Sennett, Ghandi, Fanon, Habermas, Foucault, Heintz, Wallerstein, Bourdieu, Luhmann, Galtung and many others to the phenomena of evolution, social construction, stabilization, and change or decay of power structures (McIntire, 1986).

Such generation of further knowledge in social work would have to formulate the following questions:

(1) What are possible responses to powerlessness in the context of cumulative social problems? What then is empowerment of unattractive, powerless people vis-à-vis social organizations, including social agencies using inhibiting power?

The *first* approach would be to learn to speak openly about power with clients, within our groups – not only about power outside our reach, but including the power both worker and agency have over them. A sense of helplessness in relation to society leads many social workers to underestimate their power sources. Discourse should be encouraged between group members and the worker about whether it is legitimate constraining power or illegitimate hindering power and the criteria by which the judgement is made (Staub-Bernasconi 1983). In this way both learn more about power and influence.

The *second approach* would be the examination of *power bases*, stemming from personal resources – physical strength, socio-economic as *resource power*, epistemological capacities as *articulation power*, symbolic models and means as *symbolic power*, competences as positional power or *authority*, social relations and informal as well as formal memberships as *organizational power*. The powerless can, as a rule, rely only on their bodies (strike, sit-ins, demonstrations, flight) or symbolic power (sound information, good theories, visions). Yet, power is not only what the individual, one's group or organization have, but also what others have. It could be crucial to know the social memberships and positions of an influential person, his or her visions, goals and habitual modes of problem-explanation or-solving. Such an analysis is the basis for the next important step: the decision about what to do with one's own and other's power sources. Here, social fantasy replaces analysis for the definition of gradual interventions steps. Gradual means that one starts with the imagination of a step of low energy and time consuming action and ends, perhaps, with the vision of a large national campaign or alternative project. So often, social workers do not do anything, when they diagnose power problems because they do not see the next step. The notion of steps requires an assessment of where cooperation may turn into conflict, i.e., by making things public. Then, reflection about the possible risks – for the group as well as for the worker – is needed. Empowerment means the mobilization of any power source for pursuing legitimate needs and goals.

(2) What kind of social action is possible against institutionalized unfair distribution of goods – for a fairer share of them? Unfair social stratification and distribution of goods and services is the most difficult question within our societies and world society. Yet,

there is a relatively accessible good in comparison with capital, land and income: It is education. The International "Movement of the Fourth World" puts its whole hope in education (Rosenfeld, 1989). Many social agencies and third-world organizations have determined that the crucial issue is education adapted to personal, local and regional needs and aspirations. One could even tie the problem of an assured basic income with the involvement in an educational program, which would either be very idiosyncratic (for immigrant women, old people, prison inmates, psychiatric patients, etc.) and/or offer access to better qualified work. This should raise the societal prestige of clients on relief, because of a new balance between rights and duties, and a possibility to overcome dependency, allowing for small or even large emancipation steps.

In the face of global information diffusion by satellites and satellite-universities and a new emerging gap between the information-rich and the information-poor, social work would have the task of finding access to these new means of stratification. Re-distribution of capital, land, technology, etc. may not be in the realm of social workers, yet the new distribution of knowledge for social problem solving may very well be a function of social work. Empowerment would then mean to seek access to the national and international cultural subsystems linking different (sub)cultures together in order to claim a fair share for the clients of social work.

(3) What kind of social action can be conceived against dehumanizing division of labor and social control as dominance? From social research, quite a lot is known about division of labor, social organization and control which hinder or motivate, which respect or dehumanize and exploit human beings. While the social worker may not redesign IBM, he/she can possibly redesign the division of labor, the role definitions, the control and power within families, groups and agencies, eventually communities – including client-participation in some form.

(4) What kind of actions are prone to initiate public discussion of universal and special social contracts and their values? Although power structures may be created by force or money, human history and social research show that every power elite has, in some way, to look for approval and consensus among its members. To detect and openly discuss illegitimate ideas which are at the core of domi-

nation of other races, ethnic groups, nations, women, etc. must be a special concern for social work.

Here, empowerment would mean to search for a complex notion of social justice, which doesn't mean that all have to get the same share. Such considerations can start in the classroom, when social work students try to find out how to distribute fieldwork income or fellowships according to basic needs, personal achievements and social responsibility. In Switzerland social workers had the opportunity to participate in the formulation of the constitution of a new canton, the canton of Jura. Pioneer workers asked for a better, fairer economic and political world order—including a property order which is responsive to the basic needs of all people. It might be said that this is "only symbolic power and empowerment," but according to Simone Weil all revolutions are first of a symbolic nature without knowing it! This is no *idealistic approach* to social work and social power. It is the only approach possible to those who don't dispose of the *material base*, especially socio-economic and organizational power-sources! It is the approach to those, who have to draw on knowledge about social change from the periphery.

(5) What social action can be taken against violence towards individuals, especially women and children? Social work has a long tradition of refugee work—work with victims of inhibiting power structures. A new approach has emerged in the refuge houses for battered, abused women and children. Professionals themselves may be targets of violence as representatives of a society with so many inhibiting power-structures. In most cases violence is not a natural feature or outburst of irrational men, but socially constructed by unjust social stratification, functional organization, ideological legitimation and coercion. This leads to the paradox, that if one wants to prevent violence, one has to empower people with other power-sources than bodily strength and weaponry. Isn't it this very paradox which social workers should bring into public discussion?

CONCLUSION

The writer hopes to have shown how relevant problem theory and problem centered modes of action in regard to power problems could be for social work. As a matter of fact: In today's world personal or private problems are not only public issues, but international problems are personal problems. This would call for transnational organization of clients and stronger networks for social work and social work education — a means of global empowerment in a globalized world-society.

REFERENCES

Addams, J. (1930). *Second Twenty Years at Hull House*. New York: MacMillan.

Alinsky, S. (1971). *Rules for Radicals*. New York: Random House.

Bartlett, H.M. (1976). *The Common Base of Social Work Practice*. New York: NASW.

Bunge, M. (1989). Treatise on Basic Philosophy, 8 Volumes, Vol 8: *Ethics, the Good and the Right*. Boston: Reidel.

Chess, W. A. & Norlin, J. M. (1988). *Human Behavior and the Social Environment: A Social Systems Model*. Boston: Allyn & Bacon.

Dan-Cohen, M. (1986). *Rights, Persons, and Organizations*. Berkeley: U of California.

Freire, P. (1980). *Erziehung als Praxis der Freiheit*. Hamburg: Rowohlt.

Germain, C. B. & Giterman, A. (1980). *The Life Model of Social Work Practice*. New York: Columbia U Press.

Gramson, William A. (1975). The Strategy of Social Protest. Homewood, IL: Dorsey Press.

Grosser, C. (1973). A Polemic on Advocacy: Past, Present and Future, in: Kahn, A.J. (Ed.): Shaping the New Social Work. New York: Columbia Univ. Press, pp. 77-96.

Konopka, G. 3rd Ed. 1983. *Social Group Work: A Helping Process*. Englewood Cliffs, N.J.: Prentice-Hall.

Laszlo, E. (1987). *Evolution, Contributions to the Understanding of the World Problematique*. The Club of Rome Information Series, Vol. 3. New York & Zurich: Europaverlag.

McIntire, E. L. (1986). Empowerment as an Outcome of Practice: An Examination of Theories of Power and the Relationships between Theory and Practice, *Paper presented at the 4th Intern. Symposium on Social Development of the Inter-University-Consortium for International Social Development, Tokyo*. Unpublished manuscript.

Papell, C.P. & Rothman, B.R. (1966). Social Group Work Models: Possession and Heritage. *J. of Education for Social Work* 2:66-77.

Piven, F.F. & Cloward, R.A. (1977). *Poor People's Movements*. New York: Pantheon Books.

Rosenfeld, J. M. (1989). Emergence from Extreme Poverty. The International Movement ATD Fourth World and its Work with and behalf of the Poorest Families. Paris: Science et Service Quart Monde.

Schulze, H. (1983). *Sozialarbeit in Lateinamerika. Solidarisieren — Nicht integrieren*. Munchen: AG SPAK M 53.

Schwartz, W. (1976). *Between Client and System: Mediating Function*. Roberts, R.W. & Northen, H. (Eds.): Theories of Social Work with Groups. New York: Columbia U Press, 171-197.

Staub-Bernasconi, S. (1983). *Soziale Probleme – Dimensionen ihrer Artikulation. Umrisse einer Theorie Sozialer Probleme als Beitrag zu einem theoretischen Bezugsrahmen Sozialer Arbeit*. CH-Diessenhofen: Rüegger (Ph.D.-Thesis).

Staub-Bernasconi, S. (1986). Soziale Arbeit als eine besondere Art des Umgangs mit Menschen, Ressourcen und Ideen. Zur Entwicklung einer handlungstheoretischen Wissensbasis Sozialer Arbeit. *Sozialarbeit. 18* (10) (complete issue).

Staub-Bernasconi, S. (1988). Theoretiker und PraktikerInnen Sozialer Arbeit – Essay ueber symbolische Macht und die Bewegungsgesetze des Bildungskapitals. *Schweiz, Z. f. Soziologie. 14* (3), 445-468. (English Summary in: Sociological Abstracts 1989).

Staub-Bernasconi, S. (1988a). Disparities between Local, National and International Development – the Need for New Social Contracts and New Curriculas. An Action Research Project and its Implications for the Theory of Social Work. *Paper presented at IASSW-Congress 1988. Vienna*. Unpublished manuscript.

Staub-Bernasconi, S. (1988b). Historical Overview Regarding Knowledge Base of Social Work in Europe and USA (1875-1980). LOWY L. et al. *An Assessment-Survey Report of Indigenous Social Work Literature on Social Work Methodology*. Boston: Boston U School of Social Work, 71-72.

Staub-Bernasconi, S. (1989). *Jane Addams – Pioneer Theoretician of Social Work and Her Significance for Social Work Education Today*. Fachhochschule für Sozialarbeit und Sozialpädagogik Berlin (Ed.). 60 Years International Association of Schools of Social Work. Eine Festschrift, Berlin, 27-38.

Vinter, R. (1967). *Readings in Groupwork Practice*. Ann Arbor, Mich.: Campus Publ.

Wilson G. & Ryland, G. (1949). *Social Group Work Practice – The Creative Use of Social Process*. Boston: Houghton Mifflin.

Zurich, October 15th, 1990/StB

Advocacy and Social Action: Key Elements in the Structural Approach to Direct Practice in Social Work

Gale Goldberg Wood
Ruth R. Middleman

SUMMARY. The structural approach to direct practice in social work assumes that opportunities and resources are unequally distributed and that members of deprived and vulnerable populations are social victims. Thus, the basic thrust of the social worker is to change oppressive situations instead of the people trapped in them. Disenfranchised, powerless, and oppressed people need a fairer share of basic economic and social goods. This makes advocacy a key practice role involving both work with groups of clients and with others who can make things happen for clients. The paper describes and illustrates instances of advocacy as the structurally oriented social worker applies six basic principles to help meet the needs of clients.

When problems arise in any given person-environment situation, what characterizes the structural social worker's approach is that she looks first to the environment as a possible source. The structural social worker's professional assignment involves (1) helping people connect with needed resources, (2) helping people negotiate problematic situations, and (3) changing social arrangements where the existing ones limit human functioning, and it is feasible to change them (Wood and Middleman, 1989). This assignment holds whether the limiting environment is the client's living situation or

Gale Goldberg Wood, EdD and Ruth R. Middleman, EdD, Professors, are affiliated with Kent School of Social Work, University of Louisville, Louisville, KY 40292.

the service system itself as it impacts on the worker, the client, or the worker-client transaction.

Fulfilling this professional assignment makes advocacy a key practice role, involving work with both individuals and groups of clients as well as with others who can make things happen for clients. It also involves work with colleagues and higher-ups to make good things happen in the worker's orbit.

FORMS OF ADVOCACY

The structural approach recognizes that advocacy has many forms. Because information is a potent resource, there are times when providing clients with pertinent and consequential information which they did not know empowers them to get what they need. For example, a client seeking to regain custody of her son now that she has a job is empowered by the social worker who tells her, in advance, the assessment criteria that are used to make such determinations. And there are times when giving information to workers empowers them, as when a child protective services supervisor advises workers about details of courtroom behavior that are valued by a new, sitting judge.

Another form of advocacy involves consciousness raising. Workers can help clients understand that their plight is not caused by personal deficits, which they were socialized to believe, but by a sociopolitical/economic system that devalues and limits them. Advocacy of this type is almost always needed in work with battered wives who have been taught that they are to blame for the beatings done to them. The use of the group in consciousness raising enables members to support each other's efforts to see their situation in a new and potentially liberating way, to challenge each other's "slips" back to defining their plight in terms of personal inadequacies, and to provide each other with the mutual aid essential to real empowerment (Richan, 1989).

Consciousness raising is equally important for social workers themselves, especially with respect to exposing the subtle, victim-blaming assumptions that underlie much staff training in such things as time management and stress management purported to combat burnout, where the roots of the problem exist in the stresses and ambiguities of organizational arrangements. Some organizations invest heavily in workshops and institutes for workers to learn the latest techniques and approaches which erroneously presuppose that, "if only the workers knew more, things would be better." Meanwhile, in these same organizations, staff meetings consume time with top-down directives and injunctions that could easily be put in written form. In this way, workers are made to adjust to the organization as a given. What if this time were devoted to opportunities for staff to work and think together, to devise creative ways around service blockages, ways to reduce redundancy and red tape? What if efforts were made to create conditions where the skills and knowledge that workers already have will get the chance to be used? What if workers expressed their frustrations and ideas to each other, supporting and empowering each other?

A third form of advocacy involves the social worker with the system that is withholding clients' entitlements. Often, all the worker needs to do to get the client what he needs is to describe the problem to a worker in that other system, and ask, "What can we do to get Mr. Jones a set of dentures?" Too many social workers skip this step, believing that the client would not have been refused if such a simple move on the part of the worker could result in obtaining the needed resource. Unfortunately, there are many organizations that treat social workers much better than they do clients. So there are times when it *is* this simple. Likewise, there are some instances where social workers are limited by agency practices and standard operating procedures which have come to be treated as if they were policy. Often, all that is needed here is a search of the policy manual, agency handbook, or other pertinent documents to reveal how everyday practices have developed a life of their own and have no justification in policy. This can open the door to changes in practice.

A fourth type of advocacy requires the worker to actually argue for the client's entitlement with decision-makers in a system that is not providing what it ought to provide, as when residents of a high rise for the elderly have been promised a night security guard but are not given one. In the organizational realm, supervisors often have to argue for what is in the best interests of workers, e.g., for flextime, for educational leave, for differential caseloads.

It is only in its fifth form that advocacy involves organizing clients to push for their rights *en masse*. This form of advocacy is reserved for situations in which all other forms have been tried and did not work, and should only be used after lengthy discussion with clients regarding the possible negative consequences they could incur if they choose this route and, fully aware of this, they wish to proceed anyhow.

When the worker using the fourth or fifth form of advocacy obtains the benefits due the clients, a concession has been made. From a structural perspective, this calls for an immediate shift in stance. The person who conceded must now be engaged as a partner in outrage over the violation of client rights, rather than as a defeated adversary. Not only does this shift help the other person to save face; it paves the way for cooperative action to modify or create a structure through which all present and future clients can get their needs met without requiring an advocate. For example, teenage defendants in youth detention centers often must appear in court represented by a public defender who has no knowledge of them or their situations. The defense is *pro forma*. A structure in which the spirit of the law is better carried out can be an arrangement with the Public Defender's Office for a weekly time when an attorney can meet with the teens at the detention center in advance of their hearings. For the structural social worker, the aim of advocacy is always universalistic, rather than exceptionalistic—getting this concession for this client at this time. Implicit in such universalism is the idea that every instance of advocacy is part of, must be part of, and reflects a broader ideology relating to social and economic justice and the human right of all people to live decently, whether or not they are part of the work force. In fact, the structural approach to direct practice draws its name from such work to create on-going structural arrangements.

LOOKING BEYOND THE CLIENT

An integral component of the structural approach, and a key to advocacy as well, is the mandate that the social worker look beyond the client to see if others are in the same plight. In terms of the structural approach, the outcome of the effort determines whether or not a structural change is needed. In terms of advocacy, the outcome of the effort determines whether the appropriate level is "case" or "cause," whether a particular situation needs to be changed for one person, or a change in circumstances is indicated for many.

Looking beyond the client to see if there are others in the same plight is one of the first things the social worker does. Initially, the worker hears of a problem—sometimes from one person, sometimes from several. In either event, the worker listens, reaching for and getting with feelings as needed, reaching for information and checking out inferences.

Perhaps a man confined to a wheel chair is frustrated and angry that he cannot visit his elderly parents at their nursing home in another city, despite the fact that the nursing home is directly on the route of a major intercity bus company. The problem, he says, is that the buses are not equipped with wheel chair lifts and wide doors. Or perhaps a working mother cannot find adequate, affordable day care for her three year old daughter and is worried that she may have to quit her job—thereby losing her seniority and the accompanying benefits.

Adhering to the principle that workers should make themselves accountable to their clients, the social worker, in both of the above instances, would develop an initial contract with the client, a contract to determine whether or not there are other people in the same plight. This critical step taken at the outset—looking beyond the client to see if others have the same problem—determines whether a structural change or an individual arrangement is the appropriate goal. If the man in the above example is the only disabled person wanting or needing to travel beyond the city limits, making a special arrangement for the man to go by taxi cab or with a volunteer in a private car would be the appropriate task. Similarly, if the woman is the only person who needs and cannot obtain adequate, affordable day care in her particular town, locating and arranging for a baby sitter, or obtaining financial assistance to help defray day care costs is sufficient.

If, on the other hand, there are many mothers who need day care in order to go to work, then a structural change is needed—a reasonably priced day care facility. Similarly, if there are many wheelchair-bound people seeking access to places beyond the city limits, a structural change such as having the intercity bus company equip some of its buses with wide doors and lifts is the appropriate goal.

Looking beyond the client to see if others are in a similar plight also has implications for the type of advocacy the worker ought to pursue. If no others have the same difficulty, *case* advocacy is appropriate. But if there are others with the same problem, *cause* advocacy is in order.

This distinction between case and cause is especially salient in these days of continual cutbacks in the social welfare arena. Freezes on hiring have resulted in enormous caseloads for direct practitioners, leaving little, if any, time to engage in organizing clients to take action at the political level. In such instances, when the social worker looks beyond any given client and finds others with the same need, she can log this information with organizations specifically designed to protect and promote "the political and economic interests of groups of people who have been neglected, stigmatized, or otherwise denied access to opportunities" (Patti, 1985, 9), e.g., The Children's Defense Fund, the National Organization for Women, or the American Association of Retired Persons. Over the last decade, most of the advocacy in the human services field has been done by such advocacy organizations (Reisch, 1990). The direct service worker who connects with appropriate advocacy organizations by logging relevant instances of need and injustice expands her efforts to help clients gain access to opportunities and resources (Taylor, 1987) without expanding her work hours. In doing this, she/he also adds to the advocacy organization's power base and thus the chances for broader structural change to be accomplished.

BELIEVING SOCIAL WORK CAN MAKE A DIFFERENCE

It should be noted that social work practice in general, and advocacy and social action in particular, require a belief that things can be better than they are and that it is possible to make them better (Grosser, 1973). Given eight years of Reaganomics followed by the Bush administration's dogged adherence to the same regressive policies, however, such idealism is hard to retain. Yet some do. Some social workers retain their dedication to social change and their commitment to the profession's ideals of fairness and justice. And there is evidence to suggest that those who do share three salient beliefs (Wagner, 1989). First, they consider client empowerment to be part and parcel of good social work practice, making social work a somewhat subversive activity. Second, they believe that consciousness raising on a micro-level is not only effective, but is a political and radical social change strategy. And third, they "view good social work practice as a vehicle for social change, even though it does not directly link clients to political action overtly" (Wagner, 1989, 393). In other words, social workers who remain dedicated to the profession as well as committed to social change seem to have focused on what they *could do* rather than what they could not do in the face of severe federal, state and local government cutbacks in domestic social programs, fiscal resources, and civil rights.

The idea of doing what one *can* do is consistent with the principles of the structural approach. If brokerage and mediation do not result in getting clients what they need, with client permission the social worker moves to the role of advocate. And, if all forms of advocacy in behalf of clients also fail, the worker continues to pursue social change through raising the consciousness of clients even as he or she works to create self-help/mutual-support groups to partially fill the gaps that ought not to exist. For example, the social worker with the group of wheelchair-bound clients would tell them, "Public transportation *should be* available to you; the bus company is denying you the right to inexpensive travel which it provides for those who are not disabled." To the group of mothers without access to local, affordable, day care services, the worker would say, "Reasonably priced day care *should be* available to you."

SELF-HELP/MUTUAL-SUPPORT STRUCTURES

The creation of self-help/mutual-support structures is predicated on the social worker's recognition that every client is not only a person in need. Every client is also a person with resources. It is further predicated on the assumption that social workers make it a matter of course to know what resources and strengths their clients have to offer, thereby making it possible to identify need-meeting linkages. For example, if the worker knows that an elderly man who needs some house repairs happens to be a good cook and, if that worker can identify a person capable of doing the needed work who would enjoy some good, home-cooked meals, the worker can link the people to each other, thereby creating a mutually beneficial "trade unit" (Wood and Middleman, 1989).

Trade units need not be limited to pairs of persons. Groups can be formed to help formerly battered women share apartments, child care, and support for each others' efforts to start a new life. The worker who brings them together can help them to see their plight as part of the dynamics of domination and oppression in a culture that values men more than women.

LEAST CONTEST

Another principle of structural social work practice that has implications for advocacy and social action is its principle of least contest. This principle guides the worker to use the least force necessary to accomplish the task, thereby minimizing unwanted counterforce. This principle is especially important in the process of identifying and sequencing the tasks necessary to accomplish the goal. For example, at the top of the list, there would be low threat moves such as exploratory talk with relevant decision-makers by the social worker alone, rather than by both the worker and an assemblage of those in need. The latter is a more threatening move and would be reserved for later use if less threatening moves do not succeed. At the very bottom of the list would be organized protests and media campaigns which bring unwanted negative publicity to the target organizations and finally, nuisance tactics like sit-ins that interfere with routine work. As a last resort, wheel chairs can delay buses at key intersections along their routes and large groups of angry adults walking around day care facilities can frighten parents into keeping their toddlers at home, thereby inflicting economic sanctions on day care providers who refuse to use a sliding fee scale.

Although social workers guided by the structural approach take no action whatsoever without the informed and explicit agreement of their clients, before moving with clients to any bottom-of-the-list activities, social workers have a special responsibility to raise the "other side of advocacy." Because the social worker can never guarantee a successful outcome without repercussions to those who participate in social action efforts, participants are often fraught with ambivalence, whether or not they are fully cognizant of it at the time. Excitement and anger can chase away second thoughts, second thoughts that ought sometimes to be heeded. Thus the worker has to reach for the fearful "no" behind the enthusiastic "yes." Because it is the clients who must live with the consequences, the clients must face the possibility of defeat, recognize their ambivalence, and understand that it is still possible to say "no," if that best suits them. Thus the social worker raising the other side of advocacy helps group members think specifically about the possible negative consequences to themselves of engaging in more threatening social action. And if the client group decides to push no further, the social worker must accept and abide by that decision, hard though it may be at this point in the process. But encouraging and abiding by the client's fully thought out decision speaks to the very heart of self-determination, to a genuine respect for the rights of people to decide their own destiny.

Like starting with low threat moves and gradually escalating until client need is met, all avenues have been exhausted, or clients choose to stop, the principle of least contest also suggests that social workers start their efforts to meet client need with the assumption that relevant decision-makers will appreciate the needs of clients and want to be responsive. Such an attitude can sometimes set a positive self-fulfilling prophesy in motion, to the benefit of all concerned. If this does not happen, and if one interaction after another suggests this is not the case, the social worker's original assumption of a complementarity of interest should shift to an assumption that, though the potential for a complementarity of interest probably exists, something has gotten in the way and obscures it. It is only as a last resort that the worker assumes that a conflict of interest exists and acts accordingly.

THE SELF PRINCIPLE

Thus far advocacy has been discussed within the guiding framework of the following principles: accountability to the client; looking beyond the client to see if others are in a similar plight, maximizing environmental supports, and proceeding from an assumption of least contest. Side by side with examples of the way in which these principles guide advocacy in behalf of clients, examples of their application to work in behalf of social workers themselves have also been provided. This was done because there is another principle critical to the structural approach, a principle that accents the importance of using these same principles in behalf of one's self.

The Self Principle cautions the worker against the selfless posture that is all too common in the profession. The tasks of advocacy require a worker who is self-*full*, a worker with confidence and a keen sense of her/his own power. Workers are guided by the Self Principle to actively pursue opportunities to influence their colleagues, community influentials, and the profession itself, in order to enhance their range of impact and affect organizational life for the better. For example, workers should hold colleagues and supervisors accountable for whatever has been mutually agreed upon. Workers should look beyond their own frustrations to see if others have the same problems so that professional problem-solving and support groups can be developed within the agency. Workers should confer with administrators to build in time for workshops to continue their education in areas which they target for themselves. And workers should advise and otherwise work with legislators in behalf of social work.

While it is recognized that the Self Principle is both a tall order and an unusual adjunct to practice theory, practitioners have long felt the need for such a theory-based guideline to validate and systematize what they have been doing in a covert and piecemeal way, often with much guilt they should not need to feel. Airlines tell parents with young children that in the event oxygen is needed on board, they should secure their own masks first. Why? Because someone struggling to breathe cannot adequately help others with breathing problems. Similarly, social workers trapped by bureaucratic obstacles cannot help clients get out of their traps.

CONCLUDING THOUGHTS

Social workers can be distinguished from other human service professionals. They have been educated in the historical and current aspects of sociopolitical/economic forces that systematically disadvantage certain groups of people. Their professional ancestors were politically astute activists who helped establish well baby clinics, mental hospitals, settlement houses, child labor laws, and other structural reforms. They have studied social policy and social welfare history. Person-in-situation has always been an organizing emphasis in social work and social work education so that, wherever graduates practice, they can recognize and appreciate environmental stress factors as well as personal dynamics. More than any other professionals in the health and mental health arenas, social workers use their understanding of the situation not only to have a more complete view of the client, but to do something about the situation itself.

This is not necessarily advocacy. For the most part it is brokerage to other agencies, or counseling with parents and/or partners of the client, or the whole family. Advocacy demands two additional things. First, it requires a certain political perspective. More than understanding the client's situation, it requires an understanding of the way in which the client's particular situation is connected to the broader problem of power differentials based on social class, race, gender, age and ethnicity. And second, advocacy requires courage. It is not easy to be disliked, especially when one is fighting the good fight.

REFERENCES

Grosser, Charles F. *New Directions in Community Organization: From Enabling to Advocacy*. (New York: Praeger, 1973).

Patti, Rino. "In Search of Purpose for Social Welfare Administration," *Administration in Social Work*, 9 (1985) 1-4.

Reisch, Michael. "Organizational Structure and Client Advocacy: Lessons From the 1980s," *Social Work*, 35:1 (1990) 73-74.

Richan, Willard C. "Empowering Students to Empower Others: A Community-Based Field Practicum," *Social Work Education*, 25:3 (1989) 276-283.

Taylor, Eleanor D. *From Issue to Action* (Lancaster, PA: Family and Children's Service, 1987).

Wagner, David. "Fate of Idealism in Social Work: Alternative Experiences of Professional Careers," *Social Work*, 34:5 (1989) 389-395.

Wood, Gale Goldberg, and Middleman, Ruth R. *The Structural Approach to Direct Practice in Social Work* (New York: Columbia University Press, 1989).

Barriers to Effective Social Action by Groups

Charles Garvin

SUMMARY. This paper presents an analysis of the barriers to social action in social group work. These barriers are seen as springing
from the educational, professional, organizational, and societal contexts of practice. After an examination of such barriers, solutions are
proposed. These include changes in the curricula of social work
schools, developments in practice theory, modifications in agency
conditions, and linkages to instruments of social change in the larger
society.

Since the beginning of social group work as a social work
method, its philosophy has emphasized a commitment to social
action. As Coyle stated:

> Group work may contribute to social change in essential and
> significant respects. Whether or not it will do so in practice
> will depend on whether group workers adopt *educational ob-
> jectives which recognize social needs as well as individual
> growth.* For the fulfilling of such objectives the group worker
> will require not only a set of techniques—valuable as they
> are—not only a skill in program making or in organization but,
> in addition, a social philosophy and the courage to turn his
> philosophy into action. Only so can he become an adequate
> group worker or for that matter—which is perhaps more impor-
> tant—an adequate citizen of a new age. (Coyle, 1947, p. 156)

Through the writings of Coyle and others (Klein, 1953; Grinnell
and Kyte, 1974; Vinter and Galinsky, 1985; Garvin et al., 1985)

Charles Garvin, PhD, is Professor, School of Social Work, The University of
Michigan, Ann Arbor, MI 48109-1285.

group workers have access to social action philosophy, theory, and skills. They also have been able to draw upon community organization literature which offers many approaches to social action that can be utilized in group work situations (Cox et al., 1987; Kramer and Specht, 1983). Finally, the almost universal utilization by social work writers of an ecological perspective reinforces the idea of the unity of persons *and* environments and of attention to both entities (Germain and Gitterman, 1987).

There are many practice situations in which social action would be an appropriate activity and yet it takes place only to a limited degree. We have no indication of how frequently social action does occur in social group work so this pessimistic portrayal is largely anecdotal. It would be useful to determine when social action did *not* occur, what the specific barriers had been. This does not imply that social action is always an appropriate activity. Our proposition, however, is that it is appropriate more frequently than is recognized or practiced.

This paper offers a series of propositions about the barriers to social action in social work groups. It also "jumps the gun" by proposing some ways these barriers can be removed, should they exist as widely as is assumed.

The conceptual framework utilized in considering such barriers is an ecological and systemic one in which the group and the social worker are seen as functioning in an interdependent manner with each other as well as with many other systems. Such systems include group work educational programs, professional and inter-professional associations, social agencies, and the institutions of the larger society. Many of the barriers to social action stem from the transactions among these systems. Group workers must have the courage to turn their philosophy into action because courage is necessary to confront these systemic barriers to social action.

This concept of barriers takes some (but not all) of the onus off the group worker when the group she or he works with is not engaged in social action. Part of the burden can be placed on the systemic circumstances which, at times, are the most appropriate targets for change if effective social action is to occur in the future. Consequently this paper is devoted to analyzing these circumstances.

SPECIFIC BARRIERS TO SOCIAL ACTION

The Education and Training of Group Workers

The standards governing the education of social work students require that both undergraduate as well as graduate schools prepare them to "service systems of various sizes and types" (CSWE, 1984). This implies that students should learn how to work with others to promote changes in the social environment as well as in individuals. How educators should weave these strands together is left up to each school. When the vast majority of social work students specialize in direct or clinical practice and take few courses in working to change organizations, communities, or even larger social systems, this issue is highlighted.

Direct practice courses focus much more on individual change than on working with these individuals in groups to promote social change. For example, a number of group work courses in schools of social work use Yalom (1985) as the major text. While this is a valuable resource for people working with groups, it is not one that incorporates the vision of the environmental focus of social group work. Thus, most students learn little about social action in their "micro" courses and are not likely to enroll in many "macro" courses.

There are few macro courses in the curriculum because of the few students who specialize in that level of practice. Integration of micro and macro courses is something about which most academics talk and about which very little is done. If learning includes "doing," the situation is even worse. Students who have field placements involving direct practice have negligible experience in social action. This is because field instructors have been educated in the same way as their students. Additional agency placed barriers to social action will be discussed later.

An examination of course syllabi indicates that structural factors which promote client problems are unlikely to be addressed in micro practice courses. Add the high status accorded by many students and faculty to "therapy" and the educational picture darkens even further. Even from an ideological point of view, the value issues taken up in classes are not likely to include the philosophical bases for a commitment to social action.

The Client Career

Another barrier to social action is the way individuals are referred to groups and their preparation for that experience. Psychiatrists, psychologists, and even social workers referring people to social work groups are likely to emphasize that the reason is to help them gain interpersonal skills and insights. Have we ever encountered a referral to social group work in which the referring agent explained that groups may be places to join with others to ameliorate oppressive social circumstances? If the individual even hints at that purpose, it is typically criticized as a defensive response.

A host of reasons account for this. Human services professionals primarily receive psychologically oriented education. Their concept of professional responsibility is to focus on individual functioning. The idea that this may be "blaming the victim" is foreign to them. Other professionals (and even some social workers) have usually been taught about group services through group psychotherapy literature heavily psychoanalytically oriented.

Further, the media and other popular vehicles through which individuals learn about groups are likely to portray members as typically engaged in processes of interpretation and confrontation. No wonder group members themselves are surprised when workers introduce ideas about social action.

Professional Writings and Associations

Barriers to social action result from the models of group work theory and practice utilized in papers delivered at meetings of such professional associations as the National Association of Social Workers (NASW) and the Association for the Advancement of Social Work with Groups (AASWG). An examination of these papers indicates that they offer little help to workers with reference to social action. The citations draw from psychoanalytic, behavioral, and human potential literature and the practice settings are likely to be psychiatric rather than those in which more social action takes place. The issues discussed include agency and social contexts more as vehicles for worker understanding than as targets for change.

Social group work models upon which presentations are based

frequently draw from the writings of Schwartz (1977), Vinter (1985), and others influenced by them. These authors, so different from one another, both incorporated ways of thinking about environmental change in their models. Neither emphasized the role of social action in social group work as much as those who identified with the "social goals" model (Papell and Rothman, 1966). This had an impact on what is now known as the "mainstream model" but writers who identify with that framework do not place as much stress on social action as they do on such concepts as "mutual aid" and the use of the group process (Middleman and Goldberg, 1987).

The Agency Contexts for Social Group Work Practice

Many issues with respect to a social action emphasis are posed by the nature of agency auspices for social work practice with groups. Consider the widening gap between social group work and such community agencies as settlement houses and Jewish Community Centers. These agencies, because of their closeness to community conditions, were natural environments for community oriented social action activities.

Social work with groups is now more likely to occur in other types of settings. Agencies oriented to specific problem areas such as medical, psychiatric, correctional, child welfare, and family breakdown are prone to focus on individual rather than societal change. One reason lies in the nature of funding. No medical insurance plan pays for social action! Environmental change is not usually in the coded outcome categories developed by public agencies and is, therefore, not legitimated as part of professional efforts.

One of the last major examples of public support for environmental combined with individual change efforts, was the Mobilization for Youth (Weissman, 1969) which was substantially reduced in scope by dismantling of the "War on Poverty." The history of that effort is well worth studying. The lessons it teaches may be very relevant, if and when the funding climate changes.

Agencies also influence practice in subtle ways. In many instances social workers in direct practice settings are provided with psychiatric consultation. In none are they provided with a similar resource for environmental intervention. There are few instances where workers have been criticized for being too "psychological" but many for being too social action oriented. Agencies have feared the reaction of the political power structure and funding bodies to social action because it threatens existing institutions and the way they "do business."

Conditions in the Larger Society

Group workers are well aware of the ideological and social conditions in the larger society that inhibit social action. These include the conservative political forces that seek to protect social institutions and to attribute people's problems to the individuals themselves; the weakness of many social change oriented organizations; and the lack of governmental support for change related activities.

On the other hand, there are also examples of energetic social change efforts in the hundreds of self-help organizations — many with a social action focus such as The Alliance for the Mentally Ill which is both a resource for consumers of mental health services and their families as well as a potent advocate for better services. This is also not the 1950's, when social activists were persecuted as "reds."

SOLUTIONS

In order to remove these barriers to engaging in social action, extensive changes must be brought about in the entire fabric of social group work theory and practice. These changes have serious implications for the agencies in which social group work occurs as well as for how workers and members understand and deal with large social institutions. In order to partialize this complex issue such changes are categorized in relationship to the theory and practice of social group work and how these are learned, the role of the group worker, the agency contexts of group work, interagency transactions involving group services, and societal issues confronted by workers and members.

Theory and Practice

One of the major issues faced by social work education is how to help students acquire a philosophy as well as values that will help guide practice. This issue, as it relates to support of social action, is an old one in social work and relates to early controversies as to whether the profession was oriented to a "cause" or a "function." This topic must again be seen as important for social work education with the idea of "cause" fully explored and explicated. While ecological theories provide a conceptual base, they do not offer a philosophical one having to do with a vision of persons as proactive organisms with a right to work to create better environments for human beings.

In this type of education, all courses in social group work should consider the social problems faced by group members and how the worker could help the members address them. All group work students should have course content on the ways that groups can engage in social action. In addition to including this to a significant degree in the group work curriculum, it should also be covered in required courses in methods of social change.

All students who have field assignments in social group work should have opportunities to practice the skills of helping groups engage in social action activities. These skills are also learned as students seek to change their own educational institutions. When this occurs it should be seen as a sign not only of the health of the students but of the institutions themselves.

These recommendations have implications for the models of group work that are taught. The "social goals" model should be reconceptualized in the light of contemporary theory and practice. This does not mean that other practice models should be ignored. In fact, they would be invigorated by ties to a clear sense of social purpose.

The Role of the Worker

These ideas require understanding by practitioners (shared with group members and relevant others) that the worker's role is not exclusively or even primarily that of therapist. The worker's role must be defined so that the activities of advocacy, mediation, negotiation, and brokerage are central and not peripheral. He/she should function as a helpful resource for a variety of social action skills such as the use of the media, formation of coalitions, the conduct of educational campaigns, negotiation, and confrontation.

Agency Contexts

How group workers seek to impact on agencies to enhance the use of social action by groups involves the choice of where to practice the methods to modify agency policies and procedures. More group workers should be helped to examine opportunities for employment with community agencies. This does not mean withdrawal of workers from other agencies but, rather, that community agencies offer opportunities for social action practice that can affect practice in other settings.

Current consultations between the AASWG and the associations of community centers, JCC's, and YWCA's are an important step. It is not enough, however, to pursue such interactions. The AASWG should explore the effective use of social group workers in these neighborhood agencies and make recommendations about this. Where these agencies may have lost their sense of direction, group workers can help them rediscover it. This is not to deny the vitality displayed by *some* of these agencies in meeting the needs of their communities and utilizing social workers in this process.

Examples of effective social action by agencies and their groups and members should be developed. The current healthy emphasis on empirical findings requires that the effects of social action upon both individuals and systems be documented. Such evidence must be presented to decision making and funding bodies accompanied by lobbying efforts to gain attention to the value of social action as an agency function.

The AASWG as well as group workers, educators, and practitioners skilled in social action should be available for agency consultation. The purpose is to consider the appropriateness of social action to specific situations and increase awareness by workers and agencies about opportunities for such activities. This may require external funding to demonstrate the value of such consultation.

Agencies should be helped to assess the barriers to social action in their settings. These may include political, fund raising, agency reward systems, and structural conditions. The agency should engage in problem solving to alleviate such conditions. At times this assessment can be done by the agency's staff. At other times, external resources will be required to provide the necessary leverage.

An agency's commitment to social action is related to its structure for promoting responsibility and accountability in its operation. Pinderhughes (1983) in her now classic article "Empowerment for our Clients and Ourselves," points out the clear connection between how we create better conditions for ourselves, how we learn to become empowered, and how these processes involve the consumers of social services and the professionals. The issue of greater participation by members and workers in agency policy making cannot be separated from how the agency will ultimately support social change efforts.

Interagency Transactions

The interagency arena includes interactions between service providers as well as among professional organizations, agencies, and practitioners. Other professionals need to be informed about the social action components of social group work and how these can benefit their clients. Contemporary case examples should be prepared and distributed.

Examples of inner city parents pressing for better schools; consumers of mental health services lobbying for housing, job or recreational services; prison inmates demanding a humane prison environment could be utilized in media to present an image of social group work which portrays its social action component.

The professional climate also impacts on this issue. There is and has been a bifurcation of professional organizations between the micro and the macro. Many clinically oriented social workers believe that NASW is too policy oriented and insensitive to clinical issues. This has led to creation of clinical social work societies. Overall, the professional environment provides insufficient encouragement to group workers who consider social action an important component of member problem solving.

Additionally, review committees that select papers for group work sessions should seek out papers oriented to social action in practice. Engagement by our professional organizations in social action also requires renewed emphasis. The AASWG's social action committee has been a less active component of the organization. Those members who have recently sought to move in this direction need more support.

Societal Conditions

To create a climate for change group workers and groups should form coalitions with other institutions for a "common cause." At the present time, when appropriate, alliances with the many active minority and women's organizations should be sought.

Group workers should be prepared to recognize that homeostatic forces exist in all systems and these, by definition, oppose change. It is naive to assume that a change effort will not meet with resistance. The dynamics of resistance at all levels of social organization must be anticipated and understood.

The power of a system to resist is often proportionate to the size of that system. When a small group tackles a large institution, the latter may have the capability to sustain a long and effective opposition strategy. As an example, during a rent strike the landlords were able to initiate a series of court hearings which exhausted the patience and resources of group members. This is not to argue against social action but a plea that the costs be identified and taken into account.

Members and workers can begin their engagement in small projects. Years ago it was fashionable to sneer at the frequency with which groups undertook to improve garbage collection. Yet Jane Addams was appointed to a sanitation position to which she gave as much energy as did her well known efforts to promote world peace.

Group workers need an historical as well as a macro-sociological perspective (Etzioni, 1968; Coleman, Etzioni, and Porter, 1970). The readiness of societies to support change varies over time. Group workers cannot despair when society is in a conservative phase but must use these perspectives to understand the contemporary period, act accordingly (not withdraw from social action), and prepare for the next phase. Recent events in Eastern Europe demonstrate the rapidity with which new circumstances can arise.

CONCLUSION

This brief analysis suggests some of the barriers to social action in group work that stem from educational, professional, organizational, and societal sources. Some strategies for response to these have been proposed. What is needed is an extended examination of the paper's assertions and its design to break down the barriers. We hope they contribute to the beginning of a return to the roots of social group work which requires, beyond restatement, an engagement in social action for the renewal of our commitment to social change.

REFERENCES

Coleman, J., Etzioni, A. and Porter, J. *Macrosociology: Research and Theory*. Boston: Allyn & Bacon, 1970.

Cox, F. et al., *Strategies of Community Organization: Macro Practice*. 4th ed. Itasca, Ill.: Peacock, 1987.

Coyle, G. *Group Experience and Democratic Values*. New York: Women's Press, 1947.

CSWE, *Curriculum Policy Statement*, 1984.

Etzioni, A. *The Active Society*. New York: The Free Press, 1968.

Garvin et al., "Group Work Intervention in the Social Environment," in M. Sundel et al., eds. *Individual Change Through Small Groups, 2nd ed*. New York: The Free Press, 1985, 277-293.

Germain, C.B. and Gitterman, A. "Ecological Perspective," *Encyclopedia of Social Work, 18th ed*. Vol I. Silver Spring, Md.: NASW, 1987, 488-499.

Grinnell, R. and Kyte, N. "Environmental Modification: A Study," *Social Work* 20, 2 (May, 1974), 313-318.

Klein, A. *Society, Democracy, and the Group*. New York: Whiteside, Inc., 1953.

Kramer, R. and Specht, H. eds. *Readings in Community Organization Practice, 3rd ed*. Englewood Cliffs, N.J.: Prentice-Hall, 1983.

Middleman, R. and Goldberg, G. "Social Work Practice with Groups," *Encyclopedia of Social Work, 18th ed*. Vol II. Silver Spring, Md.: NASW, 1987, 714-729.

Papell, C. and Rothman, B. "Social Group Work Models: Possession and Heritage," *Journal of Education for Social Work*. 2, 2 (Fall, 1966), 66-77.

Pinderhughes, E. "Empowerment for Our Clients and Ourselves," *Social Casework*, 64 (1983), 331-338.

Schwartz, W. "Social Group Work: The Interactionist Approach," in *Encyclopedia of Social Work*. Vol 2. New York: National Association of Social Workers, 1977, 1328-1338.

Vinter, R. and Galinsky, M. "Extragroup Relations and Approaches," in M. Sundel et al., eds. *Individual Change Through Small Groups, 2nd ed.* New York: The Free Press, 1985, 266-276.

Vinter, R. "The Essential Components to Group Work Practice," in M. Sundel et al., eds. *Individual Change Through Small Groups, 2nd ed.* New York: The Free Press, 1985.

Weissman, H. ed. *Community Development in the Mobilization for Youth Experience*. New York: Association Press, 1969.

Yalom, I. *The Theory and Practice of Group Psychotherapy, 3rd ed.* New York: Basic Books, 1985.

The Critical Role of Social Action in Empowerment Oriented Groups

Enid Opal Cox

SUMMARY. This paper discusses the contribution of social action to empowerment oriented groups. It defines an empowerment oriented practice model and the role of group work practice in such a model is reviewed. The key role social action plays in empowerment oriented groups is discussed and illustrated.

Recent discussion about empowerment has reached into almost all areas of the human services. During the 1980's a number of social welfare conferences used the word empowerment in their themes. Political figures representing conservative, liberal, and progressive-radical perspectives used the term to win support. Empowerment is equated with intra-psychic change, self-care competency, group self-help, and social action. Many authors focus their observations on one of these arenas for change. The concept of empowerment appears in social work literature as part of an overall philosophical perspective, as the goal of social work practice, as a

Enid Opal Cox, DSW, Assoc. Professor, Graduate School of Social Work, and Director of the Institute of Gerontology, University of Denver, Denver CO 80208.

guide for practice strategies, as a purpose for worker interventions. A small number of practitioners have used empowerment as the core of an overall model for social work practice. Simon (1990) states:

> Subdivisions of the profession whose leaders have been much more vocal historically in underlining the distinctiveness of their respective practice approaches than in emphasizing attributes held in common with other parts of the field — casework, casemanagement, group work, community organization, and social welfare policy — have all explicitly incorporated the concept of empowerment into the very heart of their current work and value orientation and have come to view the empowerment of clients and constituents at both the individual and collective level as a central project of the overall profession. (p. 31)

The widespread use of this term without specific definition requires that at least the basic characteristics of the empowerment model of practice be identified.

The concept of empowerment practice guiding this discussion is generally supported by Pinderhughes (1983), Cox (1988), Solomon (1976), Guiterrez (1990), Kieffer (1984), Brinker-Jenkins and Joseph (1980), and Cox and Parsons (1990). While not all of these authors attempt to develop a comprehensive model of practice which may be referred to as an empowerment oriented practice model, all contribute to its construction.

The definitions of empowerment oriented practice suggested by these authors vary somewhat. For example, Cox (1988) defines empowerment oriented interventions as those methodological approaches which mobilize consumers of service and their families and communities toward (a) self-care, (b) collective self-help, and (c) authentic involvement in the creation of a better environment including politically based social action. Guiterrez (1990) states that "empowering practice differs from many other forms of social work practice in that it proposed that the goal of effective practice is not coping or adaptation but to increase the actual power of the client or community so that action can be taken to change and prevent the problems they are facing."

Brinker-Jenkins and Joseph (1980) in their observations with respect to women's issues say "liberation . . . requires mobilization at the base. Masses of women must redefine the small spaces of their lives, taking charge of and transforming their relationships with each other and their immediate environments . . . we can then begin to build movements" (p. 36). Pinderhughes (1983) suggests that the goal of empowerment is to achieve the perception of having some power over the forces that control one's self as essential to one's mental health. Power or lack of power becomes the critical issue in people's lives (p. 331). Solomon (1976) speaks of empowerment as a process whereby persons who belong to a stigmatized social category can be assisted to develop and increase skills in the exercise of interpersonal influence and the performance of valued social roles (p. 6). All of these perceptions of empowerment in relation to practice include the need to address both the personal and political dimensions of human problems.

Other common characteristics of these authors regarding empowerment oriented practice include the critical role of consciousness raising in the empowerment process and the need to establish an egalitarian relationship between client and worker. Consciousness raising in this context implies the involvement of clients in understanding the personal and political aspects of their problems and/or oppression. Personal aspects of their problems include both the personal pain experiences involved in their status and the internalized beliefs and behaviors they may have incorporated in their daily lives which tend to reinforce their status. Social psychology findings that describe ways in which we define ourselves and our capacities by the actions and perceptions of those who surround us are useful in our understanding of negative self evaluation.

Personal action/change, interpersonal change and social action are required as part of the on-going process of consciousness raising. Critical analysis requires action and on-going analysis of outcomes of that action to understand the environment more fully. For example, much is learned about the nature of an authority system when its rules are challenged. Not only are the rules often made explicit, but the strength of the enforcement mechanism is tested and the motives and beliefs of individuals involved in the organization/structure become more evident. It is important to note that consciousness raising in the empowerment oriented model of practice becomes synonymous with assessment in traditional problem solving models of practice.

THE CRITICAL ROLE OF GROUPS
IN EMPOWERMENT ORIENTED PRACTICE

Within the larger context of an empowerment framework for practice numerous group work models have added insight into both the purpose and functioning of empowerment oriented group work. Schwartz (1980) stressed the importance of group workers assuming a holistic approach, including private troubles and public issues, with respect to perceived problems.

Lee and Swenson (1986) describe the important role of mutual aid in groups which encourage members toward self empowerment. The self-help and social support movements lent support to the theme of mutual help as a powerful tool in maintenance of mental and physical health as well as in individual struggle for self empowerment. However, traditional approaches to group work practice often focus on single function groups. For example, groups are categorized as educational, growth, socialization, task, or social action groups (Toseland and Rivas, 1984). Empowerment oriented groups do not fit easily into these descriptive categories. The basic assumption in empowerment oriented practice, that the consciousness raising process is central to self empowerment, leads to identification of the group process as the most potentially productive medium.

Galper (1980), in his explication of radical practice intervention notes: "Radical analysis understands that oppressed people internalize their oppression and that this needs to be examined if people are to become free enough to deal with oppressive forces . . . Some radical therapists have suggested that a group process is more valuable than one-to-one relationships because it encourages sharing which is crucial when people confront their sense of isolation and their responsibility for causing their own problems" (pp. 145-146). On the other hand, other empowerment theorists see a key role for group process in allowing isolated individuals to find their problems are held in common with others. One frequent and important outcome of finding "common problems" is the lessening of guilt among oppressed individuals. Blaming one's self for failures which are beyond one's control can have a disempowering effect on every aspect of one's life.

Solomon (1976) describes the possible outcome of negative valuations experienced in relationship to more powerful groups through racism, discrimination and other forms of oppressive behavior:

> — Because these families accept society's label of inferiority, they are prevented from developing such optimal personal resources as a positive self-concept or certain cognitive skills — in other instances powerlessness may be expressed in an inability to develop interpersonal or technical skills because of low self-esteem or underdeveloped cognitive skills, which in turn, are a direct consequence of interaction in an oppressive society. The final step in this vicious cycle would be a reduction of the black individual's effectiveness in performing valued social roles because of his or her lack of interpersonal and technical skills. Finally, the inability to perform valued social roles confirms and reinforces feelings of inferiority and of negative values, and the vicious circle begins again. (pp. 576-577)

Empowerment oriented workers find that participation in groups is often essential to the consciousness raising process which enables individuals to challenge and change this state of existence. Exposing the fine line between self blame and learned negative or self defeating behaviors is a task which the empowerment oriented worker often finds overwhelming. The creation of an egalitarian/partnership (working relationship), which is required for exploration of problems and behavior is difficult and time consuming. Group participation for individuals experiencing similar problems can produce critical insights more quickly than one-to-one interactions, especially with a worker who may be perceived to be an authority or even the "enemy."

Guiterrez (1990) suggests that the group context can be used for the following tasks: accepting the client's definition of the problem, identifying and building upon existing strengths, engaging (the client) in a power analysis of the client's situation, teaching specific skills, and mobilizing resources or advocacy (pp. 9-10). All of the key strategies for empowerment are enhanced when developed and implemented through the small group process because individual members can supplement each others' strengths in the accomplishment of empowerment oriented activities. The group provides a milieu for demonstration to individual members that they or others who share their same life status are able to achieve the tasks essentially without outside help. For example, when the entire group is engaged in finding resources, the group learns not only about their availability but the process of finding and accessing them.

Small groups of individuals of like status provide a medium in which members can sort out the personal from the political aspects of their problems. Empowerment groups are helpful to individuals coping with and changing the internalized aspects of oppression/powerlessness in the following ways: (1) The group as a whole, through sharing experiences, can better describe the full impact of specific problems on the members' lives and the lives of their families and friends; (2) Members who have survived or overcome aspects of powerlessness can inspire and motivate others; (3) Members who have identified beliefs and/or behaviors of their own which reinforce their own oppression (i.e., belief that they cannot learn valued skills) are incapable of achieving higher status roles, or cannot have an impact on a social service agency, can confront their peers and in so doing facilitate the consciousness raising process; (4) Groups can provide a forum in which individuals can gain increased knowledge of the political dimension of their situation, and a better understanding of the origins of the personal dimensions of their problems.

Other functions of empowerment oriented group work are: (5) Trends and patterns in the environment can more quickly be determined as the group explores that environment; (6) Group members provide mutual support with respect to clarifying and understanding the problems they face (reaffirming one's right and ability to critically examine and name the problem); (7) The group provides a medium of mutual social-emotional support for members in their struggle to cope with and bring about change in both the personal and political aspect of the problem; (8) The group serves as a site for training in skills and acquiring knowledge needed for increasing competence in all aspects of empowerment i.e., personal change or social action activities; (9) The group can take action(s) intended to bring about environmental change (i.e., sending a letter to an apartment manager/owner, a rent strike, signing a petition regarding quality of care in a health maintenance organization); (10) The group can assist group members in coping with and/or challenging the outcomes or results of the change provoking action; and (11) The group serves as a source for analysis of the meaning of the reactions resulting from its change effort (i.e., How does the reaction of the target system help the group to define more clearly the target system and the problem? What is the extent and acceptability level of the results? What strategies should be next, and what outcomes may be expected? How should group members prepare for alternative possible outcomes?, etc.).

THE SOCIAL ACTION COMPONENT OF EMPOWERMENT GROUPS

Workers with groups of oppressed persons may share, in common with traditional social work practice, a tendency to focus on personal *or* political dimensions of the problem that confronts the group. Consequently, the group process outside the context of empowerment philosophy and practice does not assure an increased sense of empowerment among participants especially in regard to the larger environment. The role of social workers in empowerment groups is to promote the construction of groups that are multi-functional in nature. The functions of these groups include mutual support, education/skills building, self-help, and social action. Much of the process of empowerment oriented groups is similar to that of traditional mutual support groups, or tasks groups.

In discussion of the group process and the impact of social action on this process, the writer will use examples from two groups. One was a group of elderly residents in a low income Single Room Occupancy Hotel (SRO), the other a group of women who were receiving public assistance from a county Department of Social Services.

The groups were both organized with an overall goal of engaging participants in an on-going self empowerment process. There was a strong emphasis on the development of the competence and knowledge levels of all members and the on-going recruitment of new members or spread of the groups' resources (new knowledge or findings about available material resources) to individuals living in the hotel or of similar circumstance in the community. The groups' empowerment orientation concentrated on the development of egalitarian relationships between the worker and the group members and among group members. Leadership was for the most part shared and assumed with respect to specific tasks dependent upon individual member's knowledge and skills. In the welfare rights group the members rotated tasks. Emphasis was placed on teaching knowledge and skills to each other rather than harboring expertise.

EXAMPLE 1. THE WELFARE SELF-HELP WOMEN'S GROUP

The worker knew a number of the group's twelve core members in her role as their caseworker. The group members lived in geographical proximity and could communicate with each other on a regular basis. The worker initially helped individual clients find resources and learn to advocate for themselves vis-à-vis the Department of Social Services and other related service and resource organizations. These individuals were encouraged to meet together for the primary purpose of discussing/solving common problems. Early meetings were spent getting acquainted, identifying problems, and seeking and sharing information about the various programs/people that effected their lives (i.e., food-stamp regulations, aid to dependent children regulations, caseworkers, school system problems, etc.). The group was able to get a small sum for supplies and find meeting space where a typewriter was available. Group members set about the task of better understanding the power structure of the Department of Social Services. They identified resource persons and invited them to meetings to explain the role of the County Commissioners, the role of the State Department of Social Services, the rules and regulations of programs, the staffing patterns of the department, etc. Individual members found and read materials of concern and shared what was learned with others. With the help of a legal aid attorney, the group began to provide information to others on assistance and offer seminars on using the welfare system to residents of a low income housing project. Group members became more and more supportive of each other in their struggle to handle personal problems by: providing consultation and moral support on difficult relationships with men, encouraging one another to handle drinking problems, sharing economic resources, providing small loans, child care or giving food and other staples to each other and sharing recreational experiences. Interests quickly spread beyond Department of Social Services concerns to schools, educational and employment opportunities, and other areas of survival concern.

Many of the women spent more than 10 or 15 hours per week with group related functions. The worker met with the group at least once a week but served primarily in the role of consultant-group member. Early in the group's activities training for social action began by learning about the power structure of the Department of Social Services, attending public meetings including Department of Social Services Advisory Council meetings, and conducting case advocacy activities which brought them into contact with officials at all levels. Group members contacted bank officials for donations to enable children of ADC clients to attend special cultural events.

These activities became more aggressive – calling County Commissioners, attending meetings as a group, organizing others to attend meetings, making official requests for increased resources, and requesting changes in the Department of Social Services became regular conduct. They also organized letter writing and telephone campaigns, circulated petitions, and set up tent housing on the court-house lawn. The group discussed strategies and reviewed the outcomes of its activities over a three years life span. Many years after the weekly meetings and social action ceased, individual members maintained a strong interpersonal support network. During the process of the group's activities most of the original members became employed, or began college and other training programs.

EXAMPLE 2. ELDERLY RESIDENTS
OF A SINGLE ROOM OCCUPANCY HOTEL

Many of the elderly residents who participated in the group were coping with mental illness, physical decline, and/or alcoholism. The project worker entered the hotel with the owner's permission and spent two months meeting with individual residents to encourage them to come to a group that would explore some of their common problems. During this time the worker helped residents find resources such as dental services, tax preparation, medicare and medicaid assistance, and transportation to medical care. The first meetings focused on introductions, and identifying common problems. Group interests and priorities were determined by the members. Members were encouraged by the worker to share problem-solving resources and became actively engaged in seeking outside resources to use and share with others. From the beginning group members also shared what they learned with other residents in the hotel and invited them to participate.

Early content in the weekly group meetings centered on issues in the hotel such as crime, lighting, meals-on-wheels delivered to the front desk but never reaching the intended recipient, and other conditions. It quickly spread to medical concerns, income, mental health, and a wide range of other issues. Group members organized an in-house crime watch system, and met with the manager to discuss other problems. They also began to communicate with the owner when the manager stated he was unable to meet some of their concerns. They identified a problem of differential rental rates and attempted to pursue an equitable adjustment (older tenants of longer residency were paying more because the buildings had deteriorated and regional rental rates had declined due to an economic down turn). The manager became suspicious and upset with the group and prohibited meetings in the building. The group moved its meeting site to a near-by cafe.

As the year progressed more and more difficulties faced by individual members (alcoholism, other threatening health and mental health conditions, death of family members, and income problems) were shared in the group. Group members reported increased contact outside the meetings, sitting up with sick members, trying to help each other cut back on alcohol, "helping through bad times" such as hallucinations, etc.

Plans for a new civic center lead to the proposed and ultimate demolition of the hotel during the second year of the program. The group was actively involved in letter writing, petitions, attendance and presentations at city council meetings, and negotiations with the Department of Social Services regarding relocation. Ultimately, the group negotiated a larger than proposed relocation allowance and managed to move to an area where the core group members and many other hotel residents lived in close proximity to each other and continued meeting along with other support activities among the network.

COMMON CHARACTERISTICS

These groups shared common characteristics of empowerment oriented groups. They were multi-purpose. Various functions occurred simultaneously with different priorities from time to time. The SRO group spent two or three meetings dealing with the death of a member and the next few weeks with strategies for engagement with the owner of the hotel. The groups were developed with a hope that they might become on-going social support networks capable of empowerment oriented activities.

Outcomes of group efforts included increased ability to better understand the problems they and others around them were experiencing, provide valuable social/emotional and tangible resource support to engage in self-education and consciousness raising activities, find and share resources, engage in social action, and use these activities for further insight and consciousness raising. There was also a strong emphasis on sharing resources found within the group and with others in their communities. The overall focus on self-help was developed to expand experience in shared leadership and individual development.

Social Action for the purpose of this paper, is the taking of collective action with the intention of changing the groups' environment. Social action was not the long term goal of these groups but rather an integral and natural outcome of the mutual problem solving process in which they engaged. Social action was not seen as the best solution to empowerment effort but as one critical part of an on-going process. The shifting emphasis in group function growing out of contacts among members and outreach to new members is an important factor in understanding the role of social action in empowerment oriented groups. Members' participation in social action was viewed as only a part of getting the job done. Self-help strategies were encouraged, and the groups planned back-up mutual support activities with respect to possible outcomes of their social action.

Participation in social action appeared to have a variety of impacts on group members. This experience often increased anger at the powerful, increased awareness of the dynamics of bureaucracies, and the strengths and weaknesses of individual actors in the target systems. One participant in the welfare self help group stated, "You forget that they (Department of Social Services officials) are just plain people until you take them on." One hotel resident observed, "I thought they had all the information and answers until we studied this thing. Now, in talking to . . . , I can see we know more about relocation than they do." In both instances, although the groups were far from achieving all their demands from the target systems, confrontations with individuals and groups composing these systems exposed the human weakness of more powerful people, and the political nature of policies and their biases.

Much of the previously unexplainable oppression felt by group participants before engaging in a social action process was demystified and gave some members a greater sense of power through increased knowledge. Group members often expressed a sense of pride at having taken part in group action, having the courage to tell more powerful people what they were thinking, or demanding their rights. The group served as a source for rehearsal of presentations and support during and after such actions.

Social action efforts in both cases tended to strengthen the cohesiveness of the group by strongly reaffirming "common issues and status." Small gains, made in better safety strategies in the hotel, change in food-stamp policy, or increase in the operating hours of a service facility utilized by the group also served to reaffirm belief in the skills and abilities of group members. Negative outcomes were a source of anger or discouragement, but the group served as a source of encouragement to refocus and transform the situation into a learning experience.

Social action led to a broader understanding of the political nature of the problem at hand. The elderly residents were unaware of the strong control of the city government over the Department of Social Services prior to their effort to change department policy regarding relocation. In the welfare self-help group challenging the Department of Social Services led to exploration of local, state, and federal relationships.

The worker's role in each group was primarily to form the group, to join the group as a resource person, and to attempt to initiate empowerment oriented processes and activities. Worker activities included: (1) Identifying potential group members, supporting and modeling to engage group members in problem identification, and seeking resources to use and to share with others, (2) Encouraging the development of a group structure to allow for the fullest possible expression of the strengths (knowledge, and skills) of all members, (3) Helping the group find resources regarding the political aspects of common problems, (4) Helping group members learn communication, mediation, and advocacy skills and other strategies which enabled members to overcome obstacles to creating and maintaining strong support networks and initiate collective action. Worker's goal was both to develop an egalitarian relationship with group members and to teach skills and knowledge which they had to contribute to other group members as well as learn from the group.

Involvement in social action by group members was critical to the process of transferring knowledge and skills because the ability to engage in such action without the help of an outside organizer can only be gained through experience. In summary, empowerment oriented group workers (Cohen, 1988), (Briton, 1989), (Guiterrez, 1990) view social action as a critical component of group process. Without this activity the effectiveness of empowerment groups would be seriously limited.

REFERENCES

Brinker-Jenkins, M. and Joseph, B. (1980). Social control and social change: Toward a feminist model of social work practice. Based on paper presented at NASW conference on social work practice in a sexist society. (1981). Faculty colloquy on women's issues. Fordham University Graduate School of Social Service.

Briton, M. (1989). Liberation theology, group work, and the right of the poor and oppressed to participate in the life of the community. *Social Work with Groups*, *12*(3).

Cohen, M.B. (1988). Notes from the field: Tenant organizing with mentally ill, formerly homeless women. *Catalyst*, *6*(2), pp. 33-37.

Cox, E.O. (1988). Empowerment of the low income elderly through group work. *Social Work with Groups*, *11*(4) pp. 111-125.

Cox, E.O. & Parsons, R.J. Reaching the Hard to Reach: An Empowerment Approach with Elders Most in Need. Unpublished paper presented at the 36th An. Mtg. of the Amer. Soc. on Aging, San Francisco, Apr. 6, 1990.

Galper, J. (1980). *Social work practice: A radical perspective*. (2nd edition). Englewood Cliffs, NJ: Prentice-Hall.

Guiterrez, L.M. (1990 March). Working with women of color: An empowerment perspective. *Social Work*, *35*(2).

Kieffer, C. (1984). Citizen empowerment: A developmental perspective. In J. Rapport, C. Swift, & R. Hess (Eds). *Studies in empowerment: Steps toward understanding and action*. New York: The Haworth Press, Inc.

Lee, J.A.B. & Swenson, C.R. (1986). The concept of mutual aid. In A. Gitterman & L. Shulman (Eds). *Mutual aid groups and the life cycle*. Itasca, IL: F.E. Peacock.

Pinderhughes, E. (1983). Empowerment: For our clients and for ourselves. *Social Casework*, *64* pp. 312-314.

Schwartz, W. (1980). Private troubles and public issues: One social work job or two? In R. Klenk & R. Ryan, *The practice of social work* (2nd edition). Belmont, CA: Wadsworth Publishing.

Simon, B.L. (1990). Rethinking empowerment. *Journal of Progressive Human Services*, *1*(1).

Solomon, B. (1976). *Black empowerment: Social work in oppressed communities*. New York: Columbia Press.

Toseland, R.W. & Rivas, R.F. (1984). *An introduction to group work practice*. New York: MacMillan Publishing.

Reflections on Social Action Practice in France

Margot Breton

SUMMARY. Social action, defined as collective action directed toward a societal end (Coyle, 1947), takes place in a social context. Studying social action in different countries and hence in different sociocultural systems can enrich knowledge and practice in this neglected area of social work. This paper looks at social action practice in post-1982 France. After a brief historical introduction, it analyzes the theoretical underpinnings of one particular model of social action which defines itself as promoting rather than assisting people. That model is illustrated in a third section, and a final section raises issues related to the model.

I. HISTORICAL BACKGROUND

The French Revolution witnessed the creation of Welfare Offices (*Bureaux de Bienfaisance*) in each *commune* (a territorial division administered by a mayor) of the country. In this way, the State (*l'Etat* — the French national government) became the provider of charitable and social services, a role previously played by the Church (Gracient, 1989). Central control of social welfare services

Margot Breton is Associate Professor, Faculty of Social Work, University of Toronto, 246 Bloor St. West, Toronto, M5S 1A1, Canada.

This paper was written in the Spring of 1990 while the author was on leave in France It would not have been possible without the help of Philippe Cholet, Centre Social, Charleville-Mézières, Anny Gracient, Centre Communal d'Action Sociale, Saint-Ouen-L'Aumone, Michel Séguier, INODEP, and especially Josiane Deveaud, Mission Locale, La Rochelle. The author is very grateful to all of them. Errors and omissions are of course the author's.

lasted nearly 200 years, until 1982 when a "decentralization" law was enacted. Responsibility for a whole series of functions was to be shared with three other levels of government (in order of decreasing size of population): the *Régional*, the *Départemental*, and the *Communal*. Two years later, the *Départements* were given responsibility for "general social action," leaving to the 36,200 *communes* the task of developing "local social action" tailored to the needs of local populations. In 1986, a law modified the social structures of the *communes*, creating Communal Centres of Social Action to replace the Welfare Offices. These Centres, public institutions of which each mayor is the president, must work:

> towards the prevention [of social problems] and towards social development in the *communes*, in close relationship to public and private institutions. . . . They have extended means and can create and administer all types of services relevant to social action. (In Gracient, 1989, pp. 3-4 — my translation)

In a research document on local social development, Séguier et al. (1987) postulate that the expansion of the roles of elected local officials in social intervention has resulted in increased knowledge and understanding on their part of what social work is all about. They document that decentralization has brought social workers and elected officials together so that their relationship is now formally conceptualized as that of "partners." However, these same researchers note that although decentralization aimed to bring relevant decision-makers closer to the local democratic process and to increase the participation of citizens in that process, it can and sometimes has led to a reinforcement of local "feudal" powers which now dispose of considerable organizational and financial means.

The new social action role of elected officials is having a profound impact on French social work. Some see in these changes a drastically reduced maneuvering space for social workers, while others welcome the necessity to tap "local solidarity" through innovative and imaginative approaches (Séguier et al., 1987).

II. A THEORETICAL BASIS FOR SOCIAL ACTION IN FRANCE

For those who take the latter view, decentralization is the occasion to revise a social work model which was ensconced in individual (case) work and traditionally oriented towards personal change. In the new model, collective work is not viewed in opposition to individual work; indeed such an opposition is identified as "manifestly outdated" (Séguier et al., 1988, p. 8), and the complementarity of individual and collective work is acknowledged. The sociopolitical and historical facts of decentralization do impose new partnerships and new roles on French social workers and lead to new ways of thinking about their practice.

One new way of thinking, that social action should "promote" rather than "assist" people, involves understanding reality "from below" rather than assuming one can do so "from above" — Saul Alinsky and Paulo Freire are recognized as prime originators of this intellectual position (Séguier et al., 1987). This is a response to the process of marginalization of groups and social classes (e.g., unskilled youths, workers in non-performing industries), rather than to the problems of marginalized individuals or families. Seeing the collective (groups or social classes) and the concrete ("from below") methodologically translates into: (a) identifying the economic, social and cultural dimensions of social action; (b) identifying all partners involved in a plan of social action; (c) identifying the various aspects of the three stages of social action — conscientization, mobilization and organization; and (d) evaluating the results of the social action.

The Economic, Social and Cultural Dimensions of Social Action

Séguier et al.'s research establishes that most often taking the economic dimension into account implies a local response to a crisis, to local unemployment for example, rather than more global social interventions. These "micro economic" responses (e.g., the creation of localized employment opportunities) constitute valuable, though limited, solutions to industrial and demographic transformations. Furthermore, dealing with economic realities can lead to new solidarities, and generate social development by creating local exchange and mutual help networks.

The social dimension of local social action involves recognizing the potentialities of the population and activating the local democratic process which requires that the information available to the population be as complete as possible. This is necessary to reinforce the abilities of citizens to take initiatives. The population then has the means to develop responsibility and initiate mutual-help approaches different from traditional assistance-giving approaches.

As for the cultural dimension, social action gives (or returns) to the population the means of appropriating its cultural identity. Thus the concept of culture, as yet defined mostly by its institutional or market aspects, may give way to a process through which the population becomes capable of defining and mastering its own mode of cultural expression and organization.

The Partners in Social Action

Five categories of partners are identified (Séguier et al., 1987) as sharing responsibility with social workers for planning and conducting social action: (1) The potential users of services who will not support social action unless it is relevant to their particular situation. They are deemed to constitute an enormous source of energy and resources. (2) The representatives of *Associations* (public or private philanthropic bodies which function as pressure groups). They defend the interests of their constituents, and thus contribute to a vibrant social fabric. (3) Elected local and departmental officials, especially local politicians who are eager to do a good job of managing their *commune* and care about what happens to its inhabitants. Having extended powers and financial means, they can play a potentially significant role in local social action. (4) "Socio-professionals." For example, banks or businesses like *restos du coeur* (literally, restaurants of the heart) which contract with a municipality to serve subsidized noon meals to senior citizens. Their input is needed to develop innovative socio-economic approaches. (5) Institutions—public administrations, specialized services (e.g., child protection agencies), schools, the media. They provide services to the local population, and their support is critical.

The Stages of Social Action: Conscientization, Mobilization, and Organization

The analyses of French social action projects consistently begin with a report of the research that preceded the actual work (Deveaud, 1989; Paquier, 1989; Rivoire, 1987; Rodier, 1987; Séguier et al., 1987; Terrien, 1987). This preparatory stage is identified as crucial. "It is before the beginning of the activity, in its conception and elaboration, that the stakes are highest. It is at this point that energy must be invested" (Séguier et al., 1987, p. 13 – my translation).

Indeed, in order to arrive at the ultimate stage of social action, when a given group (or population) organizes itself to act on a social objective, the group must have mobilized itself, i.e., must be committed and ready to participate in organizing an action. To mobilize itself for action, the group must have a sense of commonality and of solidarity with others who will be involved in or affected by the action.

Awareness of commonality and shared fate – of collective identity – cannot develop unless people have information on what they share with others and their common fate (e.g., the ecologists have made (most of) us realize that we collectively share the earth, and what happens to any part of it will eventually affect all of us). Objective information apt to produce a 'collective identity' will be more readily available if some preliminary research (e.g., population and environmental profiles, needs assessments) has been conducted. Such research identifies the common interests, values, needs, and problems of a population or social class, as well as the social partners considered to be either potential or actual allies or adversaries. Therefore the conscientization stage includes two substages: a preconsciousness-raising stage of information-gathering or research which allows the development of the consciousness-raising stage per se wherein people awake to a sense of collective identity and solidarity, as well as to an awareness of the environmental (cultural, socio-economic and political) dimensions of their situation.

Issues concerning the stages of social action include the need for better analytical tools to study the processes which allow: the development of a collective conscience leading to strategic actions; a sustained mobilization of a group or population; and efficient organizational practices. Another issue is the need to recognize both 'practical' and 'symbolic' action, the first concerned with efficiency, the second being of a festive or celebratory nature. In the dialectical processes by which the actors in a social action go from action to reflection on the action and back to action, the realization of a collective identity and the taking of collective action generate a desire to celebrate. The collective celebration is the symbolic part of social action in which the collective ownership of the action and the collective participation in its preparation and execution is celebrated. It may well be crucial to the vitality of each stage.

A third issue is the need to develop techniques and methodologies for action, including the means to mediate at various levels. Mediating involves constructing and utilizing time and spaces in such a way that at the relationship level, people interact and opinions are exchanged and confronted; at the organizational level, information circulates and actions are coordinated; at the symbolic level, collective creativity is expressed, and the discovery of a collective identity is celebrated; and, at the institutional level, relations with experts and decision makers are established, positions confronted, and negotiations and participation in decision making take place.

Evaluating the Results of the Social Action

Evaluation is discussed in terms of: (1) assessing the range of participation of the population, i.e., potential service users, from its absence to belonging to a well developed group; (2) identifying the stumbling blocks in the processes of conscientization, mobilization and organization; (3) evaluating the role(s) of the social workers; and (4) evaluating the effects produced or induced (psychosocial, socioeconomic, political).

A social science researcher (and mayor of a small town in Brittany) concluded a discussion of French social action and local development experiences by cautioning that, if these efforts are to have any long term impact: "there is no other solution but a patient and tenacious struggle of democratic renewal, starting from 'below' and finding in solidarity with other groups acting in the same direction, the means of progressively engaging all levels of power" (Houée, 1988, p. 54 — my translation).

III. A SOCIAL ACTION-ORIENTED PRACTICE

This section illustrates the preceding theoretical analysis. The example involves a summer youth employment and vacation program in the La Rochelle area of western France which lasted from 1985 to 1989 and involved a total of 93 young men and women (Deveaud, 1989). By the early 1980's, many French youth were becoming marginal to their society, principally, but not only, through economic estrangement, i.e., unemployment. A national policy to fight this marginalization gave birth in 1984 to a program of "Works of Collective Utility" (*Travaux d'Utilité Collective* or *TUC*). Public funds were allocated to local projects which, while useful to a community, aimed at reinserting youth into the economic and social life of their environment:

> The *TUC* are open to any youth aged 16 to 21, who is not working or studying full time. The youths work part-time (80 hrs/mth). The duration can vary from 3 months to a year. (Law of October 16, 1984, in Deveaud, 1989, Notes — my translation)

The La Rochelle *Mission Locale* whose objective is to ensure that youth find a professional and social place in society (this is referred to as "insertion") decided to organize a *TUC* program in the *communes* of the island of Ré (off La Rochelle) which, in the summer, becomes a major vacation resort. The work consisted of maintenance tasks associated with the arrival of tourists: upkeep of camping grounds, beaches, roads, and parks.

The objectives involved both personal and societal (structural) change. In terms of personal change, the youths contracted with social workers to learn to negotiate their status of trainees/employees with the municipalities and to cope with the various demands of that role. They also contracted to learn to manage their free time. In terms of structural change, local social systems were expected to function differently: (a) social workers assigned to various services were challenged to work together more effectively; (b) different youth serving *Associations* and institutions were challenged to coordinate their efforts; and (c) elected municipal representatives were challenged to reassess their views of, and deal differently with the problems of economically and socially marginalized youths.

The Economic, Social and Cultural Dimensions of the "TUC en ILES" (Islands TUC) Program

The economic dimension amounted to a local response to youth unemployment. The program aimed to generate local development by creating new solidarities and networks among youths, social workers, institutions, and *Associations* and between all of these and elected officials. The social dimension involved recognizing potentialities as reflected in the program objectives. Though the youths were known to have personal problems resulting from difficult family situations (immigrant parents, unemployed fathers, mothers dependent on welfare, rejections, abandonments) as well as a history of poor social adaptation (early school drop-out, gang delinquency, aimlessness), their potential for learning and changing was acknowledged. The potential of the other partners was also recognized: the professionals were assumed to be willing to form new work alliances and to relinquish previously defended 'turfs'; the *Associations* were presumed to be interested in the successful outcome of a socially useful program; the institutions were seen as capable of cooperation and coordination; and the local politicians were perceived as ready to listen to new ideas and willing to risk new long term problem-solving approaches. Activating the local democratic process was done through the use of small groups where decision making was in the hands of the members: (a) groups of 2 or 3 youth working in a particular *commune* who learned to use local resources and collectively (either in these small groups or in a larger group comprising all youth working on a given island) organize their leisure activities (at a time when worldwide many youth experience periodic unemployment or face long-term under-employment, this type of learning is not to be underrated, for it has consequences in relation not only to personal satisfaction but to the resilience of the social fabric in democratic systems); (b) a group of social workers who planned the major aspects of the program and its financing, and supported the youth throughout their experiences; (c) a group of representatives from the participating social services, *Associations*, and institutions (*groupe de Pilotage*/Piloting group) whose task was to sustain the program when it was extended to three islands, thus to the entire *département*; and finally (d) ad hoc groups of social workers and elected local politicians in which negotiations and decisions were made regarding the exact nature of the work to be done by the youth, and financial issues.

The cultural dimension was expressed in the determination of the planners to give the youth the means of appropriating their cultural identity by valuing their way of organizing and using leisure time. These youths had never set foot on the islands (though they lived close by). They perceived the life and leisure activities of the relatively well-to-do vacationers as a foreign culture. The planners challenged the youth not to be cowed by what the 'market' or others proposed as *the* way of spending vacations (e.g., sunning oneself on a beach), nor to fall back on old habits (e.g hanging out in dance halls), but to discover what they could do with the available leisure resources (such as boating and deep-sea fishing) which would feel 'right' to them.

The Partners

Four of the five categories of partners identified in the theoretical framework participated in the *TUC en ILES* program; the fifth, made up of private sector partners, could not be included by reason of a law forbidding *TUCs* to use private funds. *The youth* (or user population) were fully informed of the project, discussed the social action objectives (the creation of opportunities for short and long-term youth employment) and contracted personal objectives (learning the role of worker, learning to manage free time). *The representatives of Associations*, in this case specialized local prevention associations, participated in the management of the operation. *Elected politicians*, contacted in the early planning stages, negotiated the general conditions of work and the welcome of the youth by the municipalities with the social workers. The welcome included free accommodation in municipal camp grounds, free meals, provision of bicycles for the youngsters to travel around the islands, and remunerations for the participating social workers. Finally, *the institutions*: the public administrations, with which the social workers negotiated the overall financing of the operation, included the central government, the *Conseil Général* (or administrative institution of the *Département*), the *C.A F.* (or Family Allowances), and the *Direction Départementale de la Jeunesse et des Sports* (Departmental Bureau for Youth and Sports). Other institutions involved were the *Education Surveillée* (Supervised Education), a bureau of the Ministry of Justice (some of the youths had been through the justice system or were still on probation), the *SIVOM* (an intercommunal or special purpose authority), and last but not least, the *Direction de la Solidarité Départementale* which 'lent' an *éducatrice spécialisée* (specialized educator/social worker), Deveaud, to the *Mission Locale*.

The Stages of Social Action in the *TUC en ILES* Program

All the partners involved in the *TUC en ILES* social action program went through the stages of conscientization, mobilization and organization. For the youth, conscientization began when they responded to the planners' trust in them by believing they had the capacity to participate in the program. It developed as they progressively became aware of their capacities (for work and for managing their free time) and realized how various social, economic, political and cultural conditions affected their participation in the program and their capacities. Through the medium of small mutual-aid groups they mobilized themselves to do something about their initial unhappiness with the available leisure-time resources and organized themselves to use the resources in a way that satisfied them.

The other partners also made that first step, believing that they could adapt to the demands of the program, which in their case were to share information and work together. Conscientization grew through the experiences of participating as equals in the planning and implementation of the program. Previously, some of these partners (especially the people from the *Associations*) may have been consulted about the objectives of a program, but were not expected to work throughout its duration as partners *equally* responsible for its success.

For these partners mobilization meant sustaining their commitment to the action over a period of five years. This was done through small groups which stimulated, challenged and supported the members to renew their preparedness for action. Through these groups the partners organized themselves, arranging for information to circulate not only within but between the groups. The groups became places where opinions were exchanged and confronted: e.g., around the exclusion of one youth who, weeding the public gardens, rid them of all the prized specimens of a particular flower which is the pride of the islands. The local politician wanted him removed from the program; the Piloting group objected; the issue was sent back to the youth group to be debated there; an ad hoc group of social workers and politicians rediscussed the issue; and the youth and the politician renegotiated a contract which permitted him to get through the program successfully.

It was in the groups that actions were coordinated: e.g., the youth wanted to rent a boat to sail around the islands and visit each other; the group of social workers and the groups of youth worked together to make this possible. Finally, it was in the groups that the discovery of collective identity was celebrated: e.g., small groups of youth from one island, and then from the other islands, started meeting together, first to go to night clubs or dance halls, then to have beach parties. Later on, they organized a dinner to which they invited the social workers and all the other partners, in a restaurant they had chosen.

Evaluation of the Social Action

Evaluation of a social action oriented practice involves four aspects: the degree of participation of the population; the difficulties in terms of conscientization, mobilization, and organization; the role of social workers; and the types of changes produced.

Degrees of Participation

In the *TUC* example, the systematic use of small groups to operationalize the program meant that all individual actors or partners were anchored to some sub-part of the whole and their participation in the social action was built-in to a certain degree. This is not always the case. In workshops which the author conducted in France, social workers expressed two concerns about partnership and partners: first, that often the population was forgotten or excluded, and second, that equality between partners was rare. Generally the politicians were perceived as having more clout. However social workers themselves admitted failing to recognize others as equals, e.g., neglecting to include in a case conference front line professionals or paraprofessionals who interact frequently and closely with service users.

Difficulties of Conscientization, Mobilization, and Organization

The first difficulty encountered by the planners of the *TUC en ILES* was related to raising the consciousness of municipal politicians about the problems facing marginalized youths. These politicians were very apprehensive, and much time was spent providing information on the youth, correcting false impressions and negotiating specific tasks which would be neither so menial as to be perceived as degrading, nor so sophisticated as to set the youth up for failure — in other words, creating optimal challenges (Harter, 1978; Breton, 1985). There were difficulties with the youth (and their families) who had to be reassured that they could live for a whole summer in the unfamiliar environment of the islands. There were problems with the administrators of services who feared loss of control over the social workers going off to the islands, perhaps falling into a holiday mood. These administrators also felt threatened by the strong working relationships developing between social workers and local politicians. This required consciousness-raising regarding the nature of professional and autonomous social work practice. An important lesson was learned about the need for patience in conscientization and mobilization work. When the *TUC* program was extended to the other islands, the planners thought they would not need to take as much time on conscientization and mobilization of the local politicians and social workers. They reasoned: "The program worked elsewhere, there are no risks" (Deveaud, personal communication). They soon learned their mistake. The organization stage never went as smoothly as previously when ample time had been set aside for *all* the stages of social action.

The Role of Social Workers

The workers first had to secure financing for the program as well as tap the interest of the potential partners. Then they had to sustain the work of conscientization, mobilization and organization of all the partners. The roles of negotiator and bargainer, catalyst and supporter came to the fore. However, the idea of partnership implies an egalitarian view of roles and responsibilities. Social workers, in this scheme, cannot be defensive about professional or organizational 'turfs.' In the *TUC* case they shared with the representatives of *Associations* and institutions equally responsible roles within the Piloting group (traditionally the institutions were seen as 'above' the *Associations* and therefore as having more decision making power). The fact that all worked together as equals throughout the program was a crucial element in the success of *TUC en ILES* (Deveaud, personal communication).

There are limits to the roles social workers can play. Some of the youth did not get along with their employers, the local politicians. To mediate these relationships an intermediary accessible to each youth on a day-to-day basis and responsible for overseeing the youth's work was necessary. 'Tutors' appointed in each commune to assume this mediating role were the municipal foremen in charge of the maintenance tasks assigned to the youth. This proved an efficient solution to the problem.

Change Produced

Social action produces effects at the psychosocial, socio-economic and political levels. The *TUC* program produced psychosocial effects in the youth as they learned, in small groups, to deal with their problems, to confront, support, and encourage each other, and to facilitate each other's integration into their social environment. The socio-economic effects are determined quantitatively: in 1986, 14 youths were employed in 5 communes; by 1989, 35 youths were employed in 11 communes. In qualitative terms, some youth negotiated more interesting jobs each summer (e.g., working on tourism brochures, setting up exhibitions). A number of youth kept in touch with the *Mission Locale* after the end of the summers: some enrolled in employment programs in fields such as construction and horticulture. Others were helped to look for jobs – a number entering the work force quite rapidly.

At the political level, the municipalities learned to approach with greater understanding and sensitivity the problems of youth unemployment and marginalization. Local politicians learned to trust the capacities of the youth, and came to realize that certain 'welcoming' conditions (e.g., financial support for meals and lodging, the free use of bicycles) made a difference in the relationships of youth to their environment. Finally, the new, more equal distribution of power between various partners, forged out of their experience of working together, remains an important long-term political effect (e.g., after the TUCs were abolished in 1989, all the island communes pressured the Mission Locale to manage a youth summer employment project, but the Mission responded that it would get involved *only* if the communes emphasize social and educational objectives, and do not reduce the program to a simple employment project financially advantageous to the municipalities).

IV. DISCUSSION

The analysis of social action oriented practice in France raises a number of issues. At the heart of such practice lies the idea and the conviction that social action involves all the various segments that make up the social fabric. These segments must be seen as partners working together. The idea of partnership involves a recognition of complementarity in the pursuit of the common good. It suggests that no partner, whether social workers, the user population or others, can "go it alone" (Janchill, 1979). It also suggests that the various partners may have differing views of the common good, views which will incorporate their own particular interests. The challenge for social workers is to accept the idea of partnership and the idea that they are not the only actors interested in the common good while remaining alert to the fact that, in their defense of the interests of the poorer and more marginalized groups in the society they will find themselves in conflict with other partners—not the least with politicians who see their own interests as linked to the interests of *all* groups in the society.

Grace Coyle warned of "the problem of competing loyalties" of modern citizenship, noting the importance of the pressure group, which she identified as "the partial group" (Coyle, 1947, p. 153). The small social work group can be seen as a "partial group." Social workers have established competence in working with such groups and fostering mutual-aid or intra-group solidarity. They must now address themselves to the problem of competing loyalties and therefore of fostering solidarity with the larger world (Breton, 1990), which implies solidarity between groups that may not have identical immediate interests.

A corollary of the recognition of partnership in social action, of complementarity in the pursuit of the common good and of solidarity to the larger world, is that conscientization, mobilization and organization concern all the actors who are or need to be part of the action—not only the members of a particular "social action group," not only the potential or actual service user population. This supports an "integrated practice" in which "the target of social intervention is the whole of social problems, rather than the rehabilitation of victims of social problems alone" (Parsons, 1988, p. 417).

Social action oriented practice must lead to action. It cannot involve only conscientization. Consciousness-raising that is not followed by mobilization and organization for action may well amount to no more than a contemporary version of the development of insight. Empowerment comes from organized action on the socio-economic, cultural and political scenes which guarantees access to existing resources. It should not be confused with personal strength which can come from the intellectual/emotional action of discovery and learning which takes place with consciousness-raising.

If it is important not to confuse strength and empowerment, or personal and social action, it is also important not to be impeded by accentuating differences between task and growth groups (or contemporary variations on that theme) but to focus on the practice implications that "growth and task elements are present in all groups" (Levinson, 1973, p. 67). The personal growth that characterizes adulthood is related to action, performance, and task accomplishment. It can be argued that in social work groups, as opposed to psychotherapeutic groups, action on the personal *and* on the societal fronts must be an always present option. Getzel and Masters (1983) demonstrated the feasibility of this approach to practice in their analysis of a group of parents of homicide victims, noting: "Helping individuals and social action are intimately connected at every turn of the group" (p. 91). These parents worked sometimes simultaneously, sometimes successively on their (personal) mourning tasks and on structural reforms (societal tasks) in the criminal justice system. Just as in the *TUC* example, meeting both personal and societal objectives was recognized as essential. Therefore, it may be more appropriate for social workers to conceptualize all their practice as personal change *and* social action oriented, instead of deciding to work *either* with "social action" groups *or* with "personal change" groups.

REFERENCES

Breton, M., "Reaching and Engaging People: Issues and Practice Principles." *Social Work With Groups*, 8: 3 (Fall, 1985), 7-21.

Breton, M., "Learning from Social Group Work Traditions." *Social Work With Groups*, 13: 3 (Fall, 1990).

Coyle, G.L. *Group Experiences and Democratic Values*. New York: Women's Press, 1947.

Deveaud, J., "Actions de Groupe *TUC en Iles* Ré-Oleron-Aix." Paper presented to the 11th Symposium on Social Work with Groups, Montréal. 1989.

Getzel, J.S. and Masters, R., "Group Work With Parents of Homicide Victims." *Social Work With Groups*, 6: 2 (Summer, 1983), 81-92.

Gracient, A., "Travail Social de Groupe et Maintien à leur Domicile des Personnes Agées." Paper presented to the 11th Symposium on Social Work with Groups, Montréal, 1989.

Harter, S., "Effectance Motivation Reconsidered: Toward a Developmental Model." *Human Development*, 21 (1978), 34-64.

Houée, P., "Les Trois Phases du Développement Endogène." In *Développement Social Local*. M. Séguier et al., Mouvement pour le Développement Social Local Poitou Charentes, 1987.

Janchill, Sister M.P., "People Cannot Go It Alone." In C.B. Germain (Ed.),

Social Work Prectice: People and Environments. New York: Columbia University Press, 1979.

Levinson, H.M., "Use and Misuse of Groups." *Social Work* (January, 1973), 66-73.

Paquier, P., "Société et Travail de Groupe: Maintien à leur Domicile des Personnes Agées et/ou Polyhandicapées." Paper presented to the 11th Symposium on Social Work with Groups, Montréal, 1989.

Parsons, R.J., Hernandez, S.H., and Jorgensen, J.D., "Integrated Practice: A Framework for Problem Solving." *Social Work* (September/October, 1988), 417-421.

Rivoire, J.M., "Traces de Décentralisation Visibles dans la Drome." *Traces*, No. 4, Mai, 1987.

Rodier, F., "Décentralisationde l'Action Sanitaire et Sociale dans le Puy-de-Dome: Jeux et Stratégies des Acteurs Principaux." *Traces*, No. 4, Mai, 1987.

Séguier, M. et al., *Développement Social Local: Une Pratique Sociale Réinventée.* Mouvement pour le Développement Social Local Poitou Charentes, 1987.

Terrien, E., "Pour la Mobilisation du Service Social, des Stratégies Possibles." *Traces*, No. 4, Mai, 1987.

Some Aspects of Empowerment: A Case Study of Work with Disadvantaged Youth

Eamonn Keenan
John Pinkerton

SUMMARY. This article describes and comments on negotiations between an agency worker, his supervisors, and a group of disadvantaged young people on the involvement of young people in the appointment of a new agency worker. It provides some background on the actors and the agency, tells what happened and aims to identify some aspects of empowerment through the use of a simple grid.

By comparison with the daily experience of disadvantage of the young people involved it is a minor experience in empowerment. Despite that it is a case study placed within a radical tradition espousing the pursuit of social justice.

Empowerment if not widely accepted, is, at least, recognised by most welfare professionals in Britain. The theme of the 1989 Annual Conference of the British Association of Social Workers was: "Empowerment and Opportunity." For the authors empowerment expresses a value base, a process and an outcome in our work with social action groups.

Living in the North of Ireland with its tradition of violent political rhetoric engenders both suspicion of sloganizing and conviction

Eamonn Keenan, CQSW. Dip. Y & CW, works in the Northern Ireland based Youth Unit of Save the Children, one of Britain's oldest voluntary child welfare organisations. He is an experienced social action groupworker, working with structurally disadvantaged young people. John Pinkerton, BSSc, MSSc, MSc, CQSW, is a social work lecturer in Queens University Belfast.

Address correspondence to either author at Department of Social Studies, Queens University, Belfast BT7 1NN, Northern Ireland.

109

about the power of words. Accordingly we need to be clear about the meaning of empowerment. For some time we have explored the practice detail of empowerment (Keenan and Pinkerton, 1988).

This paper continues this work with a case study of empowerment. It describes the negotiations between an agency worker, his supervisors, and a group of disadvantaged young people leading to their involvement in the appointment of a new agency worker. It provides background detail on the actors and the agency, tells what happened, and identifies key aspects of an empowering experience.

THE ACTORS AND THE AGENCY

The worker involved in the negotiations was Eamonn. He is professional qualified in both youth work and social work but does not define his practice primarily by identification with either occupation. In part because of his own background of socio-economic deprivation, his work is an expression of a value commitment to social justice. He works to challenge discrimination against young people through applying Freire's notion of "conscientization" (Freire, 1980). His practice is informed by such British youthwork writers as Smith (1981), Davis (1988), and Ward and Mullender (Ward, 1982, Mullender and Ward, 1985, 1988, 1989). Central to his work with young people is the view expressed by Ward that for social action groupworkers:

> The key task is to create opportunities for choice which mean something to the young people themselves . . . . The achievement of the task will entail such young people achieving and exercising power in order to bring about changes. This is best achieved collectively.

The young people are six women aged eighteen to twenty who comprise the Twinbrook Youth Action Group (T.Y.A.G.). They are a natural peer group living in Twinbrook, a large public housing estate on the outskirts of Catholic West Belfast. Northern Ireland is notorious for its poverty and political instability, by both British and European Community standards. (Harbison, 1989, Teague, 1987). Twinbrook is one of the most disadvantaged parts of this disadvantaged region. A survey (Blackman et al., 1987) revealed unemployment rates of forty seven percent for men and eighteen percent for women. Nearly a quarter of all adults live in households of six or more. Thirty percent of women have had five or more pregnancies and, some eighty five percent of children live in poverty. The politics of the estate are predominantly Irish nationalist. It is constantly patrolled by the police and the British army and has experienced countless incidents of IRA 'armed struggle.'

Given the socio-economic context and the T.Y.A.G.'s aim to identify and address issues for change in the lives of its members, it is no surprise that their primary concern is to find ways of dealing with what they regard as a masculine and repressive culture and community.

Eamonn works for Save the Children Fund (S.C.F.) one of Britain's oldest child care organisations. His involvement with the T.Y.A.G. is an expression of the agency's moves to realign its work more explicitly on the side of the powerless. Its present policy direction is built on the value base of its founder, and on its many years of practice experience in Britain and the Third World. A recent policy document states:

"The Fund is committed to working with people, not for people; to empower not control" (S.C.F., 1989, p. 2). In reviewing its work with disadvantaged young people in Britain the Fund identified them as "one of the most needy, the most vulnerable and the least powerful groups in the U.K. today" (S.C.F., 1989, p. 18).

Applying the empowerment principle to work with this group the organisation committed itself to "develop both the social action and personal development methods of work. Social action is an approach used with young people on issues and agendas that they have identified as important if they are to achieve change in their situation or environment. Personal development work aims to enable individual young people to achieve personal change by increasing their awareness, skills and knowledge" (S.C.F., 1989, p. 18).

These policy commitments are expressed through S.C.F.'s development of projects such as the Belfast based Youth Unit from which Eamonn works with the T.Y.A.G. As a project worker he is supervised by the Unit's Project Leader who is an experienced worker with a personal commitment to a participatory style of leadership. The Project Leader is directed by a manager who encourages open dialogue and challenges workers to be innovative in their practice. All these individuals and members of the T.Y.A.G. have important parts in this case study of empowerment through negotiations.

NEGOTIATING THE YOUNG PEOPLE'S INVOLVEMENT

In 1989 staff at the Youth Unit were formally advised that agency funding was available to employ a new worker. After the closing date for applications project team members conducted a review which resulted in a long list of candidates for management approval. The team were aware of and committed to the procedural implications of the interview process with respect to the agency's equal opportunities policy. They were also aware that, as a matter of policy, users, i.e., young adults, were expected to become involved in the management of projects. However, while there was an acceptance of this policy in principle, no definitive procedures had been created to implement it in the recruitment process.

The Project Leader and his manager finalised the list of applicants, and agreed on a panel of professionals and managers for the interviews which would be held over two days. This information was shared with project staff.

At this point the "first key choice" occurred. Presented with the information about the interviews, the Project Worker decided to register his surprise and disappointment at what was proposed. He asked the Project Leader when and how young people were to be involved in the interview process. He was told that, while this had been discussed by the Project Leader and his supervisor, no decision had been made.

By affirming his commitment to the direct involvement of young people in decision making and expressing his difference with management's decision the Project Worker opened a "second key choice"—not, this time, for himself but for his supervisor. The Project Leader recognised the difference between agency policy and the proposal. He went back to the manager with the conflict and asked for changes in the interview procedure. The manager recognised the difference and accepted that they had the responsibility and power to do something about it. Recognition of the need to align their actual practice with agency policy led to a commitment to change the interview procedure to accommodate the involvement of young people in the process. At the same time there were limits set on the form this could take based on the Fund's requirement to adhere to internal practices and equal opportunities policy.

Acceptance of the involvement of young people required identification of who they should be. This question was put to the Youth Unit.

Staff were asked to explore this with the young people involved. This provided the "third key choice point" – a choice not for the worker or his supervisors but for young people, including the T.Y.A.G. They were asked if they would take part in selecting a new staff member for similar work to that done by their worker but elsewhere in Belfast. They chose, with considerable enthusiasm, to be involved.

Thus three "key choices," the first by the worker, the second by his supervisor, and the third by the group of young people, were required to shift the young people's role in the appointment of a new agency worker from passive exclusion to one of active involvement. When the T.Y.A.G. chose to be involved in the interview procedure concern was expressed about what this involvement would entail. After discussion it became clear to the young people, the Project Worker, and the Project Leader that just to slot one of the young people into the existing arrangements would be tokenism. The interview procedure needed to be radically changed in a way that made it accessible to the young people as a group. Instead of a single interview with each candidate it was decided by the managers that a three stage process was needed.

First, there was to be an information night for the prospective job applicants. Included in the programme were four young people involved with the Unit, three members from the T.Y.A.G., and a young man who had been referred to the Unit for his criminal activities.

They were asked to be involved because their experience represented the two different practice approaches used by the Unit – "personal development" work with individual young criminal offenders and "social action" work with groups of young people.

Two from the T.Y.A.G. chose the task of giving a presentation about their group and their view of the agency's involvement with them.

The second stage involved preliminary interviewing to select a short list of four candidates. The interview panel was to be made up of the agency manager, project leader, and two of the young people who had taken part in the information night. These were the young man with experience of the Unit's individual approach and one of the T.Y.A.G. During the information night the two assumed listening and observing roles. They were also chosen for the practical reason that both were unemployed and available for day time interviews.

The third and final stage of selection involved interviews with those applicants who had been shortlisted. These interviews were to be conducted by senior S.C.F. staff, a member of the agency's advisory committee and a representative from another organisation. Management thought it not possible to have a young person on the final interview panel. However to insure that their earlier involvement was not seen as mere tokenism, all candidates had to have the unanimous approval of the panel to meet criteria for selection for the final interview.

PREPARATION FOR INTERVIEWS

With the changes in the interview structure the young people agreed with the project worker to prepare for their various roles in the interview process. Prior to the information night and the first interviews the young people arranged two preparatory sessions, one with the worker and one with the Project Leader. These involved planning and organising what they would say, why they would say it and how it would be said.

In the first session an exercise was conducted to identify the qualities the young people felt were important in a worker. To achieve this the project worker needed to clarify the purpose of the session and find an appropriate means for the group to do its work. He started with a statement about how he and the agency believed young people had valid and necessary knowledge and opinions regarding the sort of person who should be working with young people like themselves. That was why young people were to be on the interview panel. What he needed from them was a statement of those qualities and skills they as young people judged a worker should have, and also of those attitudes and behaviors they regarded as unhelpful or inappropriate.

This clear statement of rationale and purpose was followed by a brainstorming exercise. The outline of their worker was traced onto a large sheet of paper, and titled "Our Ideal Youth Worker." Words and comments such as "good head on shoulders," "not boring—very important," "sex of worker not important" and "not afraid to nag or push" were added by the group. The active generating of ideas grounded in the young people's own experience with their project worker created a dialogue among them and between them and the worker. The worker prompted the group with questions; "Do you want the worker to be someone who will make decisions for you?" "What if the worker was Gay?" This helped clarify and highlight the points the young people wanted to make. While the task was taken seriously, the process was generally light-hearted. Comments such as "no nose pickers" both provoked laughter and prompted discussion of the importance that the group attached to acceptable levels of personal hygiene and good manners.

At that meeting the group also wrote a script, divided work tasks and rehearsed for the presentation about the T.Y.A.G. to prospective applicants. The worker asked questions and expressed support, but offered no answers and made no decisions.

The second session was held after the information night and before the first interviews. This involved the Project Leader who supplied information about agency policies and procedures. Discussion focused on two questions, "what do we need to find out about the people being interviewed?" and "what questions do we want to ask?" The key areas that emerged related to skills, experience, values, attitudes, suitability, and readiness.

THE INTERVIEWS AND THEIR IMPACT

Three candidates met the selection criteria to progress to the second set of interviews. There was a unanimous decision about each candidate and the young people were fully involved and influential. In one case a manager was ambivalent about his reaction to an applicant. Trying to be neutral and fair, he ignored his "gut feeling" about how the candidate would get on with young people. In contrast both young people were definite in their views and able to argue successfully that the candidate's unsuitability for the post was clearly related to the criteria established.

Both young people found the process difficult for them, though they felt they were able to contribute. "I said what I wanted to say, but was afraid of being one-sided."

They attributed their nervousness to the importance of the decisions they were helping to make about adults' abilities and suitability for employment, the novelty of asking questions in a formal setting, and their feeling of inadequacy beside people who seemed experienced and comfortable with the business of interviewing. However, being taken seriously, having a clear role, and finding encouragement and support in actively participating in the process gave them confidence and helped them relax.

Almost all interviewees said they had never been interviewed by young people before and reacted positively to the idea. Project staff who did not participate in the interviews did not feel excluded and affirmed the value of putting policy into practice.

The effect on the other adults in the interview panel was important. Both were impressed by the way the young people had taken part in a mature and responsible manner. Both felt that the young people had participated at a level equal to or better than any adults with whom they had served previously. As a result of this experience the agency's Personnel Department responded positively to the manager's request that one of the young people be a full member of the final selection panel. It was recognised that this represented one way an administrative department could translate principle into practice. In the final selection process the young person felt she was competent to contribute and was in agreement with the other members of the panel about the candidate who was selected.

EMPOWERMENT AS REPOSITIONING

Empowerment is a process that draws together a range of actors and generates its own momentum involving real choices about whether to engage or not to engage. It makes heavy demands in practical and resource costs for agencies and workers.

Empowerment is not simply about the distribution of a commodity called power, which requires diminishing the stock held by some individuals or groups in order to add to that held by others. Although that may be the outcome in certain situations, in this case study empowerment is a process entailing the repositioning of social actors in their power relationships.

Empowerment as repositioning can be illustrated in more detail by returning to the three "key choices":

1. Project worker seeks involvement of young people
2. Project Leader resolves conflict between policy and practice
3. Young people decide to participate.

At each of these choice points the actors were positioned in powerful or powerless situations in relation to the appointment of the worker. The extent to which the actors felt comfortable with their situation also impacted on these choices.

These choices can be analysed using a grid (See Figure 1) made up of a horizontal plane relating to degree of power (powerless/ powerful), and a vertical plane relating to degree of acceptability, (acceptable/unacceptable). This creates four quadrants (A, B, C and D) in which it is possible to locate the key actors of the story at each of the "choice points." At each point the impact of these decisions alters the relationships, creating dilemmas to be resolved and opportunities to be grasped.

First Key Choice

Project worker seeks involvement of young people (Fig 2i & ii)

Before the first key choice (Figure 2.i), the young people (YP) are deep in Quadrant A (Acceptable Powerlessness). They are unaware of and uninvolved in the situation. The Project Leader (PL) in contrast, is deep in Quadrant B (Acceptable Powerfulness). He regards himself as actively fulfilling a management task congruent with how he sees his role and which he assumes to be legitimate.

The Project Worker (PW) is in Quadrant C (Unacceptable Powerfulness) because he regards the arrangements for the interview as unacceptable. His dilemma is pointed up by his interface position which involves him in direct relationship with both the Project

FIGURE 1. Power/Acceptability Grid

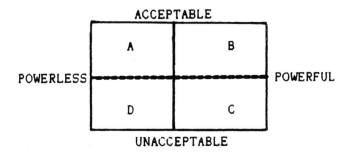

KEY :

Quadrants

A = Acceptable Powerlessness

B = Acceptable Powerfulness

C = Unacceptable Powerfulness

D = Unacceptable Powerlessness

Leader and the young people. He is powerful because of confidence in his competence as a practitioner, his effective working relationship with the Project Leader, and his knowledge about agency policy which endorses his practice ideology.

Thus the Project Worker (PW) is in the position to choose to be a creative change agent. He performed this function by questioning the Project Leader (PL) in reference to agency policy. As the legitimacy of the worker's question was recognised, the Project Leader became uncomfortable with his original approach to the interviews. This created a reversal in the positions of the Project Worker (PW) and the Project Leader (PL), (see Fig. 2.ii), The Project Worker (PW) moved to Quadrant B and the Project Leader to Quadrant C. No change has occurred in the young people's (YP) position. They continued to be unaware and uninvolved in any power play.

FIGURE 2 i & ii

2 i Before First Key Choice   2 ii After First Key Choice

A Y.P	B P.L	A Y.P	B P.W
P.W	C	P.L	C
D		D	

Second Key Choice

Project leader resolves conflict between policy and practice (Fig. 3).

The Project Leader (PL) then chose to be a creative change agent by successfully renegotiating the interview procedures with his supervisor. The result of this choice moved the Project Leader (PL) to Quadrant B (Acceptable Powerfulness) alongside the worker (PW), (Fig. 3). The young people (YP) are still in their position in Quadrant A (Acceptable Powerlessness).

Third Key Choice

Young people decide to participate (Fig 4 i & ii)

The young people (YP) agreed to become involved, which moves them into Quadrant C (Unacceptable Powerfulness) positioning them to choose a creative change agent role (Fig. 4i). The Project Leader (PL) and Project Worker (PW) remain in the powerful Quadrant B (Acceptable Powerfulness).

The young people's agreement increased their power but emphasised their lack of experience and skill in such situations hence their discomfort about their powerfulness. They (YP) now occupy the position of creative change agent. In alliance with the worker (PW),

FIGURE 3. Second Key Choice

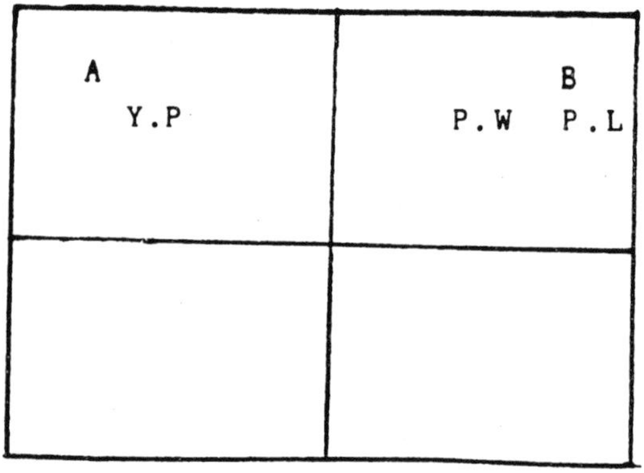

A Y . P	B P . W P . L

FIGURE 4 i & ii

Fig 4i Third Key Choice

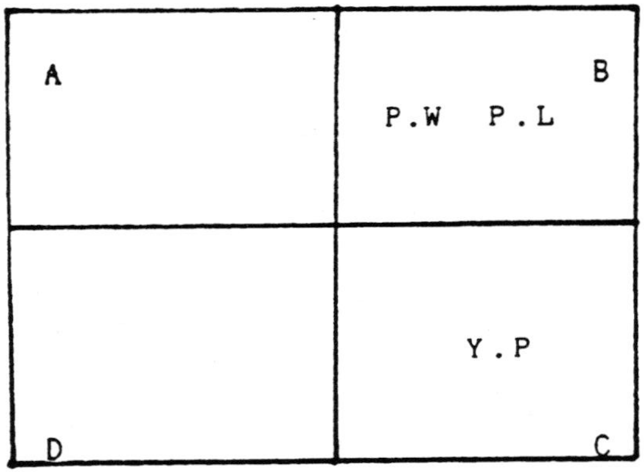

4 ii After Preperation for

Interview

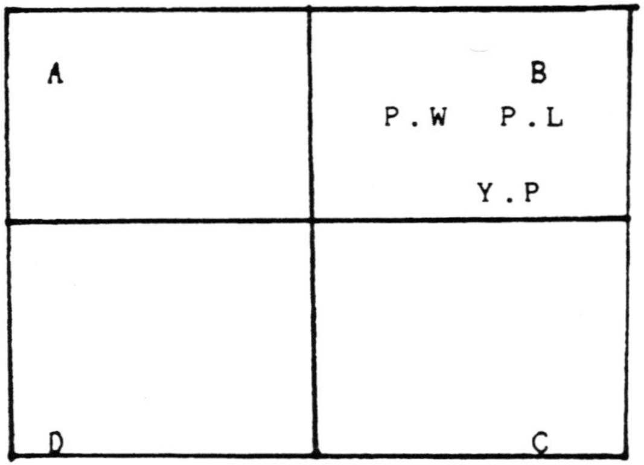

through their questioning, preparation, and involvement in the process they moved into Quadrant B (Acceptable Powerfulness) (Fig 4.ii).

Thus all of the main actors were in Quadrant B, but this was not the final point at the time of the interviews. That position can be seen in Fig. 5.

Since only one member of the T.Y.A.G. participated in the interviews, only that young person (One YP) and the Project Leader (PL) are in Quadrant B (Acceptable Powerfulness).

The other members (Other YP) and the worker (PW) have moved to Quadrant A (Acceptable Powerlessness). This is qualitatively different from their original position because they are now informed, aware of and involved in the situation.

ASPECTS OF EMPOWERMENT

From these moves across the Quadrants three important points about the process of empowerment emerge.

First, we have identified how individuals took responsibility in making their own choices creating opportunities for empowerment. The agency structure was open to challenge on the basis of its own policies and was flexible enough to change procedures. However,

FIGURE 5. Final Positions

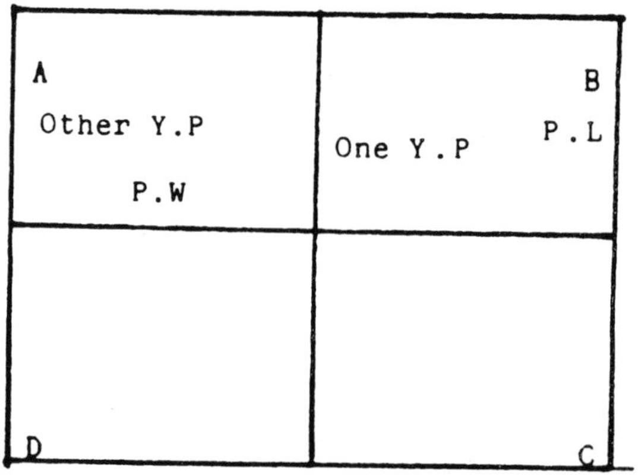

to ensure that openness and flexibility persists requires both organisational and individual forms of monitoring and vigilance.

Second, although Quadrant B (Acceptable Powerfulness) is the optimum position for exercising power and is the desired end place for those being empowered, it is actually Quadrant C (Unacceptable Powerfulness) that contains the maximum capacity for creative change.

Third, note the movement of the project worker from Unacceptable through Acceptable Powerfulness to Acceptable Powerlessness. Empowerment is neither a matter of the worker offering power in heroic alliance with service users or giving up power to users in an act of cathartic altruism. Rather, it requires that the worker confront him/herself with his/her values and power to become sufficiently uncomfortable to use that power to generate empowering choices for others. The worker must be prepared to step back as others make their own choices from the opportunities that he/she has helped to generate. Our illustration shows these choices do not necessarily, in the first instance, belong to the service user but rather are worker and management choices internal to the agency.

CONCLUSION

We have tried to describe and understand an example of empowerment. It is a mundane example because of the focus on the nuts and bolts of the process and, by comparison to the T.Y.A. Group's daily experience of disadvantage, it is a minor experience in empowerment.

Empowerment means neither taking power on other people's behalf nor disclaiming our own power in the vain hope that others will somehow benefit from our self induced powerlessness. Rather, empowerment for social action group workers means using the power of our skills, agency position or personal authority to ensure less powerful users of our services opportunities for choices. So approached, empowerment ceases to be pure rhetoric and becomes a means to engage workers, management and users in negotiating choices that are small celebrations of human dignity and democracy.

REFERENCES

Blackman, T., Evanson, E., Melaugh, M., & Woods, R. (1987). *Housing and Health in West Belfast: A Preliminary Report To The Divis Joint Development Committee.* University of Ulster.

Davis, B. (1981). *Restructuring Youth Policies in Britain – The State We're In.* Occasional Paper 21. Leicester. National Youth Bureau.

Freire, P. (1972). *Pedagogy of the Oppressed.* London. Penguin.

Harbison, J. (Ed.). (1989). *Growing Up in Northern Ireland.* Belfast. Stranmillis College. Learning Resources Unit.

Keenan, E., & Pinkerton, J. (1988). Social Action Groupwork as Negotiation: Contradictions in the Process of Empowerment. *Groupwork, 3.* pp 229-238.

Mullender, A. & Ward, D. (1985). Towards an Alternative Model of Social Groupwork. *British Journal of Social Work 15.* pp 155-172.

Mullender, A., & Ward, D. (1988). *New Horizons: Empowerment through Social Action Group Work.* Paper presented at the 10th Annual Symposium of the Association for the Advancement of Social Work with Groups. Baltimore, MD.

Mullender, A., & Ward, D. (1989). Challenging Familiar Assumptions: Preparing For and Initiating a Self-Directed group. *Groupwork 2.* pp 5-26.

Save the Children Fund. (1989). *UK Department: Policy Statement.* Unpublished paper.

Smith, M. (1981). *Creators Not Consumers.* Leicester: National Association of Youth Clubs.

Teague, P. (Ed.). (1987). *Beyond the Rhetoric – Politics, the Economy and Social Policy in Northern Ireland.* London. Lawrence and Wishart.

Ward, D. (1982). *Give 'em a Break: Social Action by Young People at Risk and in Trouble.* pp 6. Leicester. National Youth Bureau.

Empowerment Through Social Action Group Work: The 'Self-Directed' Approach

Audrey Mullender
David Ward

SUMMARY. This paper explores a particular approach to English social action group work which concentrates on goals set by members themselves to achieve external change. The key features and stages of this approach are outlined and its value-base is emphasized. Three examples of groups which reached three discrete stages of development employing the approach are presented.

Over recent years we have been involved in developing and researching an approach to work with groups aimed at empowering them to define and meet their own needs. We call this 'self-directed group work' (Mullender and Ward, 1985, pp. 163-164).

In our view, too much of conventional British group work places the entire burden of change on the client. Unintentionally, therefore, it clings to pathological explanations of behaviour and 'blames the victims' of social and economic processes which, in fact, lie outside their control (Ryan, 1971). Certainly individuals do sometimes need to change but, this change must not, by default, be wrapped up in pathology or blame. Instead, practice should be based on an understanding that the social structure, the way particular societies are organised and their norms and institutions are the source of much of human suffering. Besides this, practice needs to

Audrey Mullender is Lecturer and David Ward is Senior Lecturer in Social Work at the University of Nottingham, NG7 2RD, England. They come from backgrounds in the public Social Services and the Probation Service respectively. Both have co-led groups using the self-directed approach.

125

flow from group members' own recognition of how social institutions and socially constructed attitudes inhibit their opportunities in life. Our experience accords with the findings of those sociologists (Hall and Jefferson, 1976) whose research has shown how those at the bottom of society's pecking order have it in their power to see the world as it really is.

To work in these terms means attempting to bridge the gap between group members as individuals and wider social institutions: that is between private troubles and public issues (Wright Mills, 1970). This involves a simultaneous concern but affords primary attention to the way in which public issues penetrate private troubles (Longres and McLeod, 1980, p. 271-272). When these connections have been made explicit people can begin to break out of the guilt and despair brought about by accepting blame for problems which are not of their own making. They can then begin to experience their own power and project their energies outwards to bring about change in external factors.

Group work directed to the process of social change has a secondary advantage of achieving personal change and empowerment for group members who can experience the potential for taking control of their own lives.

In practice, this means emphasizing the members' own definitions of their situation, facilitating their understanding and working uncompromisingly with issues as they define them. Without this, there can be no awareness of wider constraints and processes, and no moving beyond members blaming themselves for their problems towards raised consciousness and the pursuit of rights and empowerment. To omit this would be to collude with processes in which explanations of and responsibility for problems are sought in the private worlds around the individual members, and knowledge and skill for bringing about change are left to those who 'know' — the professionals. These are definitions and processes which service users frequently find themselves powerless to resist and come to take for granted.

Working on these premises brings our values to the fore. This, in turn, has important consequences for our development of group work theory.

A VALUE-BASED APPROACH – PRINCIPLES FOR PRACTICE

Our work is grounded in the rich diversity of settings and responses which form the context of contemporary group work practice. These need to be nurtured and protected if group workers are to be both creative and proactive in the rapidly changing and increasingly hostile world confronting many group members. However, at the center of such fertile diversity lies a range of concepts which deserve more attention or debate than they have received up to now: the differing values, or "world views" (Papell, 1987), which explicitly or implicitly underpin the various group work approaches. These world views are insufficiently emphasised in conventional accounts of group work theory (e.g., Douglas, 1976; Papell & Rothman, 1980; Brown, 1986).

Certainly, rigorous analysis and theoretical model-building are required to discipline practice (Papell and Rothman, 1980, p. 7). Jeffs and Smith graphically state the reason:

> Students and field workers alike struggle to make sense of their practice and career on a diet of ill-digested material culled from the 'vox pop' end of sociology, social policy and psychology and a host of 'practical guides' based on folk wisdom and often little else. (1987, p. 5)

However, intellectual rigor and the confidence which it can inspire need not come from obscuring values, as is too often the case in both the American and British literature. If values are given due recognition at the core of intervention (Mullender and Ward, 1985), diversity in practice can be transposed from undisciplined eclecticism into a dynamic and refined approach which can withstand sustained evaluation. Elsewhere (Mullender and Ward, 1988), we have examined the interlinked and interdependent process of practice (action) and research (evaluation) by which this can happen.

At the heart of our value position lies the conviction, tested in practice with a range of client groups, that social action groups have an inherent capacity for bringing about social change and, with this, personal betterment and empowerment. This value position can be expressed in the following practice principles:

1. We need to take a view of the people with whom we work which refuses to accept negative labels and recognises that all people have skills, understanding and ability.
2. People have rights, including the right to be heard and the right to control their own lives. It follows that they also have the right to choose what kinds of intervention to accept in their lives. Service users must always be given the right to decide whether or not to participate in self-directed work, and the right to define issues and act on them.
3. The problems service users face are complex and can never be fully understood if they are seen solely as a result of personal inadequacies. Issues of oppression, social policy, the environment and the economy are, more often than not, and particularly in the lives of service users, major contributory forces. Practice should reflect this understanding.
4. Effective practice can be built on the knowledge that people acting collectively can be powerful. People who lack power can gain it through working together in groups.
5. All our work must challenge oppression whether by reason of race, gender, sexual orientation, age, class, disability, or any other form of social differentiation upon which spurious notions of superiority and inferiority have historically been (and continue to be) built and kept in place by the exercise of power.
6. Practise what you preach: methods of work must reflect non-elitist principles. The worker does not 'lead' the group but facilitates decision making and responsibility for and control of outcomes. Though special skills and knowledge are employed, these do not accord privilege and are not the sole province of the worker.

WORKERS AS FACILITATORS

Workers must want to work with people and not direct intervention "to" or "at" them. The group worker should find his or her most effective contribution in facilitation rather than leadership in the traditional sense. Workers using this approach assist the group to find the means to achieve its desired ends, but do not dictate what those ends should be. They make suggestions and offer alternative scenarios for consideration but their chief contribution will be to free and highlight group process, not in directing the group's work or its outcome.

Opening themselves up to hearing what service users are saying, empowering them to set their own goals, and take collective action, involves drawing out the best from group members and helping them determine where they want the group to go, rather than imposing one's own agenda on them. The worker can have a hard job explaining and maintaining this in the group. Members are used to professionals as authority figures and as providers or withholders of resources. Consequently, they expect the worker to tell them what to do and how to do it and to procure everything the group needs to make it function. It takes frequent direct explanation and practical demonstration for group members to recognise that they can look to the worker for help but not for direction. Workers have initially to be directive about being non-directive.

Often, workers unfamiliar with the role of facilitator fall into the trap of going too far and becoming totally non-interventive. Non-interventive does not mean falling over backwards to keep one's self and one's views invisible and unheard. It means playing an active role – for example, in challenging the fatalism members often bring to a new group ("There's nothing we can do about it") – yet being sensitive to the differences between keeping issues in play and dominating. In view of the subtle judgements involved, there is no less skill in this kind of work than in group work where the worker is the central figure.

Self-directed group work is a skilled activity which can be acquired and improved by careful evaluation of intervention with a consultant or supervisor experienced in the use of the approach.

KEY FEATURES AND STAGES OF THE SELF-DIRECTED GROUP WORK APPROACH

These practice principles and worker role provide a distinctive approach. Self-directed group work has its roots in direct practice. It developed as a result of working in and studying a range of groups – two of which we instituted ourselves and others which were established quite independently by practitioners in a diversity of settings and amongst a variety of client groups such as children in care, parents accused of abusing their children, disabled adults, ex-psychiatric patients, battered women, elderly people in residential care, and young offenders.

In addition to the clarity of the workers' values and role, all these groups had certain other features in common. These were their voluntary, open, non-recruited, and often large membership, their open-ended and typically long time scales, and the way in which members were encouraged to set their own goals for change, based on a collective understanding of the problems they all had in common. All were primarily directed towards seeking external change, both in attitudes and in policy and practice (Mullender and Ward, 1989).

We were struck by the difference between these key features and those which Brown et al. (1982) outline as characteristic of mainstream British group work:

> a discrete type of practice whose general features include: individual centered aims consistent with meeting client need and carrying out agency function; an eclectic theoretical base; an overall approach which values peer sharing and mutual feedback; the creative use of a range of group techniques; co-leadership; a closed membership of six to twelve adults (usually strangers initially, but sharing similar problems) and time-limited duration.'' (p. 589)

Self-directed groups normally have at least two workers. The ability to co-work effectively, often across professional boundaries, is, therefore, a fundamental skill in self-directed group work. Beyond the advantages of co-working shared with other forms of group work (Brown, 1986; Hodge, 1985), we would add a further benefit. Workers can assist one another in putting their values into operation and in holding to anti-oppressive ways of working. Published accounts of projects (Badham, 1989; Mistry, 1989) have stressed the importance of co-workers jointly developing coherent practice which incorporates an anti-racist perspective. A larger group may need more than two workers and, to ensure that it remains empowering for all, workers need to be attentive to group process at a level of concentration which fewer workers might find it hard to maintain.

In examining the self-directed approach, we identified a process through which such groups pass. It falls into three stages, each with a number of steps. The first is one of preparation in which the workers spend time reaching agreement about the values which motivate their practice. This is the point at which they choose to work along self-directed lines, opt for an alternative model, or decide that they do not constitute a compatible worker team. The second and third stages take the group through making and evaluating its own decisions about action aimed at external social change.

The ten steps of the basic three-stage model are:

Stage One: Taking Stock

a. The workers begin by formulating a coherent value position along the lines of the practice principles outlined earlier. They accept empowerment of service users as a valid aim to be pursued by addressing structural issues in day-to-day practice. The workers consider potential group members to have strengths, skills and understanding. They see them as having the ability to do things for themselves through the group and something to offer one another.

b. Once the workers have reached agreement on these matters, they can invite people who share a particular structural problem to choose to join the group. Group members become partners with the worker team in seeking solutions to wider social problems.

Stage Two: Taking Action

The group moves from recognition to action as it is helped to explore the questions 'WHAT,' 'WHY,' and 'HOW.'

c. The workers facilitate the group in setting its own agenda of issues: ASKING THE QUESTION – 'WHAT?'

d. The workers help the group to analyse why the problems on its agenda exist: ASKING THE QUESTION – 'WHY?'

e. The workers enable members to decide what actions to take. (Workers do not impose their own ideas for action, except to say they will not do certain things such as working towards racist goals.) The group members share the tasks. ASKING THE QUESTION – 'HOW?'
f. The members take those actions for themselves.

Stages (c) to (f) may recur several times during the 'Taking Action' stage.

Stage Three: Taking Over

The group is helped to perceive the connections between 'WHAT?,' 'WHY?' and 'HOW?'

g. The group reviews what it has achieved.
h. The group identifies new issues to be tackled: REFORMU-LATING 'WHAT?'
i. The group perceives the links between the different issues tackled: REFORMULATING 'WHY?'
j. The group decides what actions to take next: REFORMULAT-ING 'HOW?'

Steps (g) to (j) become a recurring process for the life of the group. Group members gradually gain some control over their own lives and realise that they have a right to more. They are now active in tackling the roots of their own oppression. In Stage Three, the workers have moved into the background.

PRACTICE EXAMPLES

The three practice examples which follow represent a wide range of clients and a diversity of ethnic origins. Some of the members faced recently acquired difficulties while others had deeply en-trenched problems. All the examples focus on workers handing over power to group members. They also demonstrate self-directed group work reaching out beyond the members' own personal coping resources to the achievement of social change on a small, localised scale. The groups all shared aims extending well beyond this. These groups reached either the first, second or third stages of the model.

Group Example One:
Rowland Dale Group for Parents
Accused of Physically Abusing Their Children

The Rowland Dale Group (Rogowski and McGrath, 1986; Mullender, 1990) was formed for the specific purpose of working in a new way. It arose from one worker's theoretical understanding of the problems facing group members and his ideological wish to pursue that understanding in his practice. Hence, the objective of the group was to focus on the physical abuse of children, not at the intra-psychic (personal stress or inadequacy) or inter-personal (family dynamics and relationships) levels, but on the structural pressures he believed featured heavily in causation. This involved:

- Attention to issues such as unemployment, poverty, and bad housing.
- Examination of the responses by statutory agencies to reports of child abuse, including formal procedures such as case conferences, and pressing for greater parental involvement in them.
- Encouraging mutual support among members during and between meetings and tapping into members' own strengths to break down the isolation and loneliness that many felt.

The Rowland Dale Group did not fully depart from traditional assumptions about group work. It did not allow members enough time to explore or arrive at their own definition of their situation or to begin to spell out or act on external goals for themselves. His original idea of encouraging its members to take over the group after the designated ten sessions was just not feasible in the time available. After six group meetings operated independently by the members, the group disbanded.

The Rowland Dale Group represents only the first stage of the self-directed model. Nevertheless, what it did achieve was a radical departure from the traditional approaches to the understanding and 'treatment' of child physical abuse, and recognition that group work can provide a way to engage the structural factors which play an important role in causation. However, the worker's role was less oriented to the self-directed approach and still largely that of the process "leader." Consequently group members were not facilitated to run the group themselves. Values represented in our first five principles cannot be expressed in practice unless the worker's role (principle six) changes accordingly.

Group Example Two: Asian Society

In response to an urgent call from the local public library to "do something" about a group of Asian young people who were "hanging around" and causing a nuisance, a team of two Asian youth workers met with the students at the nearby college. The students used the library for study but also treated it as something of a social center where they could meet friends of both sexes because its educational connotations meant their parents did not object to their going there. They felt they needed to hold meetings of Asian young people at the college, but that neither staff nor the other students would support them.

With the help of the workers, the group set goals for itself and acted to achieve them. It successfully negotiated for a place to meet at the college during normal hours. By asking itself why its interests had previously been ignored it also saw the need to confront the issue of underlying racism. It raised a number of concerns with the college authorities, including racist attacks by white students, the prejudice embedded in staff attitudes, and the organisation of the college. The Asian workers were able to use their understanding of the group members' ethnic background to assist them to explore how, as young people living in Britain, they wanted to meet their friends more freely while how, as Asian young people, they did not want to flout their families' wishes nor the cultural and religious norms of their community.

A further issue, arising from the process within the group, was the tension between the male and female members. The latter felt the young men did not listen to them, and insisted that sexism was as much a problem as racism. After withdrawing to discuss their needs on their own, the young women returned with a set of proposals which the group eventually accepted. It was decided that, when the male student social worker left, the remaining male worker would be joined by a female colleague. The group could then be assisted to review its achievements and decide what other work it needed to undertake as its "third stage" of development.

Group Example Three:
Ainsley Teenage Action Group (ATAG)

This started as a natural group of teenagers who had "offended" together in the neighbourhood where they lived. Their probation officer, along with two other workers, decided that a self-directed approach would help the young people work to improve neighbourhood leisure facilities — the lack of which had been, in their own view, an important causative factor in their offences. The teenagers wanted to recruit friends and the workers agreed, recognizing that they faced the same external problems, that it was a false distinction to see pathology in some but not others. This is in contrast to traditional group work with offenders, where workers select the members for the group, and the group is then closed.

The workers established themselves as trustworthy and reliable presences in the lives of the young people. They worked on the principles of self-direction refusing, for example, to accept members' negative labels but sought their own definitions of the problem they faced. They were committed to group action on these problems. They respected and affirmed what the young people brought to the group, encouraged them to find their own strengths, and make their own decisions.

For the group to become self-directing, it was necessary to create an informal setting in which the members felt comfortable and confident, where there was a relaxed attitude on the one hand, and as much participation as possible on the other, without undue control by the workers. Being used to being told what to do, members found it hard to discipline themselves and to manage their own meetings.

The use of structured exercises, suggested by the workers and accepted by the group, helped but was by no means the whole answer. Eventually, a system for managing these problems emerged naturally. The members came to allow themselves a wilder "relax" session at the beginning of each meeting, before getting down to "business." This became an accepted part of the meeting routine. One member said, "When we meet at the club, the first half hour we just sit around, have a drink and a general chat between ourselves. Then we get down to sorting out how we can get one step closer to getting a youth club and any paper work that needs doing. Any leaflets for handing out we'll do them at the club."

The workers discovered that in these informal sessions a lot of "business" was sorted out among the young people themselves, often pulling together discussions that had taken place outside club meetings, on the street or at school. After this, the business sessions were productive — sharp and decisive. The workers had to recognise and accept that, on occasion, the members took decisions independently and without their awareness. They needed to tune into the wavelength of this informal but powerful decision-making process whereby members might reach their own conclusions and not feel the need to communicate to them. This really tested the workers in their determination to facilitate the group in owning its own decisions and goals.

The workers encouraged the young people to explore the issues involved. By questioning the group they attempted to get the young people to examine why they felt bored. The workers also asked them to look at the implications of their offending. Who really loses out in the long run? Out of these, a plan of action emerged: what needed to be changed and how to go about achieving it.

The members produced a petition, ran a public meeting, raised funds and approached local elected representatives concerning the needs of their neighbourhood. The young people used the media and their own purposeful activities to challenge the labels of "delinquent" and "disruptive" which they had previously borne. In this way, they began to be taken seriously. By following the "What," "Why," "How," process, the workers had placed responsibility on group members, both for decisions and for action. They became increasingly able to accept this responsibility and eventually obtained a plot of land for a youth club, a portable building and a grant for essential services such as electricity and plumbing.

The group went on to review its efforts and to take up other issues, as indicated in the later stages of the self-directed group work model. One such was that of policing practices. The young people felt harassed by the police patrolling their neighbourhood. They sought and obtained a meeting with the local Chief Inspector, who agreed to put different officers on duty in return for a guarantee of a less obstructive attitude. This negotiated arrangement was kept. The Chief Inspector has since obtained equipment for the group, spoken favorably about it in a televised interview, and generally become one of the group's firmest supporters.

The group moved on to new issues and analysis of underlying injustices towards young people – particularly those in trouble with the police. They perceived that it was their status as teenagers which brought them unfair treatment, and built this awareness into their campaigning. In relation to the management of the youth club which they worked so hard to obtain, they insisted on control by young people, despite bureaucratic regulations which required adult supervision.

By this stage, two of the three workers had ceased to be involved. The remaining one saw himself in a supportive role, essentially as a consultant, helping the group take stock of its performance and move forward if it got stuck.

A postscript on social action group work in Nottingham is that the parliamentary Select Committee on Children invited another group which had links to ATAG, to meet with members of both Houses of Parliament. The young people's "consumer opinion" was confidently offered and well received.

FINDING A PLACE IN PRACTICE FOR SELF-DIRECTED GROUP WORK

Group workers have the scope to practice in ways which liberate rather than stigmatize. There is a strong tendency, however, for practitioners to assume that persuading their agencies to allow them to develop self-directed group work will be prohibitively difficult.

The practice examples we have cited illustrate that the self-directed approach can be used in a wide range of settings and contexts which could have amounted to nothing more than 'containment' or 'surveillance,' i.e., with young people on court orders (Ainsley) and parents accused of child abuse (Rowland Dale).

Self-directed group work affords the opportunity to draw on the values and skills more commonly employed by community workers — in facilitating people to take action on their own behalf. As a distinctive approach, we have firmly located it in social work agencies, involving the specialized settings of those agencies, the people who are selectively identified as social work clients and the tasks for which social workers often have formal and legal responsibility. Thus, the membership of self-directed groups and their location mark important distinctions from community work. Yet the scope which such groups offer for social change is equal to anything seen in community-based action.

As a consequence, we no longer find acceptable intervention which stops short at focusing problems onto the individual. The social worker should at least seek to follow individual work with an offer of involvement in a group — the opportunity of working towards real change, to achieve what they and their clients would ideally want and can accomplish.

There is nothing super-human about the Rowland Dale parents, the Asian college students or the Ainsley young people. Rather, social action, through self-directed group work, empowered them to find their true selves and to attain more of their real potential through tackling external, structural problems on their own terms.

REFERENCES

Badham B. (ed.), (1989), "Doing something with our lives when we're inside." Self-directive (sic) group work in a youth custody centre. *Group work*, Vol. 2(1) pp. 27-35.

Brown A., 1986, *Group work* (2nd ed.), London, Heinemann.

Brown A. & Caddick B., 1986, "Models of Social Group work in Britain: a Further Note." *British Journal of Social Work*, Vol. 16, pp. 99-103.

Brown A., Caddick B., Gardiner M. & Sleeman S., 1982, "Towards a British Model of Group work," *British Journal of Social Work*. Vol. 12. pp 587-603.

Douglas T., 1976, *Group work Practice*, London, Tavistock.

Hall S. & Jefferson T., 1976. *Resistance through Rituals*, London, Hutchinson.

Hodge F.J.B. (John), (1985), *Planning for Co-leadership: A Practice guide for Group workers*, 43 Fern Avenue, Newcastle upon Tyne, England: Groupvine.

Jeffs T. & Smith M. (eds.), 1987, *Youth Work*, London, Macmillan.

Longres J.F. & McLeod E., 1980, "Consciousness Raising and Social Work Practice," *Social Casework*, May 1980, pp. 267-276.

Mistry T., (1989), "Establishing a feminist model of group work in the probation service" *Group work*, Vol. 2 (2) pp. 145-158.

Mullender A., 1990, "Group work as a response to a structural analysis of child abuse," *Children in Society*, Vol. 3(4), pp. 345-362.

Mullender A. & Ward D., 1985, "Towards an Alternative Model of Social Group work," *British Journal of Social Work*. Vol. 15, pp. 155-172.

Mullender A. & Ward D., 1988, "What is Practice-led Research into Group work?," in Wedge P. (ed.), *Social Work—A Third Look at Research into Practice*, Birmingham (U.K.), British Association of Social Workers.

Mullender A. & Ward D., 1989, "Challenging familiar assumptions: preparing for and initiating a self-directed group," *Group work*, Vol. 2(1), pp. 5-26.

Papell C., (1987), *Group work with New Populations*, Invitational Paper presented at the Plenary Session of the 9th Annual Symposium on the Advancement of Social Work with Groups, Boston.

Papell C. & Rothman B., 1980, " Relating the Mainstream Model of Social Work with Groups to Group Psychotherapy and the Structured Group Approach," *Social Work with Groups*, Vol. 3(2), pp. 5-23.

Papell C. & Rothman B., 1988, *Social Group Work: Mainstream Model and Instructional Methods*. Paper presented at the International Congress of Schools of Social Work, Vienna.

Rogowski S. & McGrath M., 1986, "United we stand up to pressures that lead to abuse," *Social Work Today*, Vol.17 (37), May 26, pp. 13-14.

Ryan W., 1971, *Blaming the Victim*, London, Orbach & Chambers.

Ward D. & Mullender A., 1988, "The Centrality of Values in Social Work Education," *Issues in Social Work Education*, Vol. 8(1), pp. 46-54.

Wright Mills C., 1970, *The Sociological Imagination*, Harmondsworth, Penguin.

The Role of Structure in Effective Agency Advocacy

Eleanor D. Taylor

SUMMARY. Structured accountability at every agency level is essential for effective advocacy. The Lancaster model illustrates this. The structure requires commitment to the advocacy issue, clear role definition for staff, board and community members, mandated involvement of staff, board and community members (clients, professionals and people who have experienced the problem), and documentation and evaluation throughout the process.

At a time when homelessness, AIDS, affordable housing and day care for children and the aged are critical issues, agencies are increasingly engaged in active advocacy for social change.

Human service organizations require effective structures through which advocacy issues can be processed when they come to the attention of staff and board members. Where there is no structure to deal with social action, such concerns may be talked about, but little, if anything, will be done. Advocacy will not be successful on an ad hoc basis. If the agency makes a policy decision to fund its advocacy efforts, it must decide what structure will work best in its own community. Advocacy will not be pursued within the agency when no one is responsible for it. A director of advocacy is required to manage and monitor the process within which advocacy is performed, as well as stimulate board and staff to recognize and accept their role and responsibility to speak out on urgent issues for and with individuals and families.

Resistance to advocating is a common deterrent to developing advocacy as a specific agency function. Resistance may come from board members, agency staff or the executive. In Lancaster the ex-

Eleanor D. Taylor, MSW, is Director of Advocacy at Family Service, 630 Janet Ave., Lancaster, PA 17601.

ecutive introduced the idea and worked closely with a board-staff committee to determine the desirability and feasibility of an advocacy role. He helped committee members work through their resistance as they designed a structure they felt could work in the agency. The Board agreed to a trial period and has supported it ever since. Some staff members were eager to launch the effort, though some resisted. A workshop to orient board and staff members to advocacy goals, structure and possible issues demonstrated the value of working together on issues that were important to the agency's mission. The first project involved organizing a community coalition that obtained a shelter for abused women (an innovative venture in 1975). This success convinced staff of the value of agency advocacy to help their clients and brought positive recognition from the community and United Way.

Resistance to what is new and untried is normal. Fear of the untried must be understood, diagnosed and dealt with. For some the thought of initiating an advocacy function or advocating in the community raises "red flags." Advocacy does not need to do this. It can work by a careful education process or dialogue that recognizes the opposition's objections or reservations. If the study of the issue and the system is done well and the strategy is carefully planned, negotiation to a "win-win" solution can take place.

Another deterrent is obtaining financial support, but advocacy's cost efficiency can convince funders. Over time advocacy has a multiplier effect: advocacy to set up new programs or remedy dysfunctional services has a beneficial effect not only on those served currently but for uncounted people in the future.

The discussion that follows regarding the Lancaster model shows how accountability and involvement of the board can make staff and board members feel comfortable about being activist.

The advocacy structure must be accountable and involve input from every level of the agency in its decision-making and operation. In this way advocacy becomes integrated into the agency's total functioning and serves as a resource to which administration, line staff and board members can refer issues. Professionals and citizens in the community can also bring advocacy issues to the attention of the agency.

Advocacy must not only be accountable internally but also to the community. No agency can advocate in isolation; the advocacy effort must involve community professionals and people experiencing the problems about which it is advocating. When the agency feels confident in its advocacy process, this empowers others in the community to join with it.

Accountability requires the advocacy group to do its homework — to study and research. Advocacy cannot stop there. It must go on to the final test of accountability — action aimed at results. The Lancaster Family Service Advocacy structure illustrates the translation of agency commitment to social action (Figure 1).

THE LANCASTER FAMILY SERVICE MODEL

The Flow Chart for Issues shows how an advocacy issue is recorded on a "log" (Taylor, 1987). The issue, identified by a client, group or citizen, must be a problem that is known to affect many people. It is logged by either a staff or a board member. The director of advocacy circulates it to staff for comments, then to the Advocacy Committee. This standing committee of the Board reviews the log and any staff input and determines whether it meets the following agency criteria for advocacy issues: Does it meet the goals of the agency and the Advocacy function? Does the agency have expertise on the issue? Is this a critical issue impacting families currently? Will there be staff, board and community people to deal with it? What are the risks to families if nothing is done? If the Advocacy Committee chooses this issue, it requests permission from the Board to set up a Study-Action Team (SAT).

The Board considers the Advocacy Committee's recommendation and, if approved, authorizes the Committee to set up the SAT. When the SAT has completed its study and action plan, it will return to the Advocacy Committee which reports to the Board for sanction to proceed with its action plan. Upon completion of the action phase, the SAT presents a final written report to the Advocacy Committee which shares it with the Board.

Two advocacy efforts illustrate the structure within which the process operates. The first was the coalition, HOMELink, advocating for the homeless and the prevention of homelessness, which grew out of the advocacy director's initiative; the second was the Single Parent Advocacy Network (SPAN). This became an advocacy group after six people at the agency's annual meeting re-

FIGURE 1. Flow Chart for Advocacy Issues

ISSUE

↓

ADVOCACY LOG

↓

DIRECTOR OF ADVOCACY

↓

STAFF

(Review and comment on log report)

↓

ADVOCACY COMMITTEE

(Selects issue for a Study-Action Team)

↓

BOARD

(Approval sought)

↓

STUDY-ACTION TEAM

(Reports to Advocacy Committee:
1. After Study and proposed Action Plan completed.
2. After Action (or if the focus of the action changes from that originally proposed).
3. When SAT is inactive.
4. When SAT writes final report.)

↓

ADVOCACY COMMITTEE

(Reports to Board at each stage as above)

↓

BOARD

↓

DIRECTOR OF ADVOCACY

(Prepares Annual Advocacy Report)

↓

ADVOCACY EVALUATION SUBCOMMITTEE

(Annual Report plus Findings and Recommendations of the Evaluation Subcommittee)

↓

ADVOCACY COMMITTEE

↓

BOARD

sponded to a speaker's challenge that communities need to provide more support for single parents.

HOMELink. By 1984 the problem of homelessness was becoming more obvious in the Lancaster community. Since Family Service is located in a suburb of Lancaster, homeless people were not coming to its door. However, the agency could impact on homelessness through its advocacy role.

The initial log described the many aspects of homelessness and called for study of the homeless situation in Lancaster City and County. The log also suggested development of a local coalition of those knowledgeable about the homeless with the goal of joining with others statewide. The Advocacy Committee and then the Board approved setting up the Study Action Team on the Homeless in December, 1984.

A small SAT composed of a board member, the director of advocacy, and several community members who were working directly with the homeless met to outline the initial study phase. A series of fact-finding steps were recommended: (1) organize a meeting of agencies working with the homeless to find out who the homeless were, why they were homeless and what was being done to help them; (2) visit shelters and interview the homeless; (3) prepare a report of the findings; (4) share the report with the original inter-agency group as well as with others concerned about the problem; (5) develop an action plan arising out of the recommendations of the study.

A large provider meeting was held to document the problems homeless people face and what the participants felt should be done. A number of key providers offered to work on the SAT. Visits were made to all local shelters and to areas of inadequate housing. A questionnaire to obtain statistics and characteristics of the homeless was distributed to all who provided shelter to homeless persons. Shelter staff members interviewed each homeless person in their shelter to get direct information. Analysis of the information from the provider meeting and the questionnaires enabled the SAT to write the "Homeless in Lancaster County, PA" report, which contained findings and recommendations on how to help the homeless and prevent homelessness.

The SAT's Action Plan was to reach out to 500 churches and relevant agencies in the community to ask their help to work on the issue and to sensitize them to the problems of the homeless by sharing the report's recommendations. This action plan was approved by the Board.

Eighty people responded to the invitation to come to a meeting prepared to work on one of the recommendations for action in the report. As a result seven subcommittees were formed to work on various tasks: low income housing, emergency housing funds, budget counseling, information and resources for discharged prisoners, preparation of a brochure on surviving on a welfare grant, advocacy for the mentally ill homeless, and publicity. The SAT became a community network with the logo HOMELink.

All subcommittees reported to a steering committee on a monthly basis. These subcommittees remained working advocacy groups until 1989 when five were spun off to existing agencies. This made it possible to refocus energies on consciousness-raising and advocacy for low income housing. Key events for the public were: a meeting at which eleven homeless people told legislators and 300 citizens what it is like to be homeless, a countywide affordable housing conference to learn about models used elsewhere in the country, and a "No Room at the Inn" Tour through shelters and public housing to see the magnitude of the problem and that public housing can be a "good neighbor."

By 1990 the United Way put together a partnership of banks, government, and non-profits to develop housing known as Partners for Affordable Housing on which HOMELink was asked to serve. Currently, HOMELink is bringing together several community and church groups who want to enable or build low income housing. HOMELink plans to seek independent non-profit status, funding, and staff. While maintaining its advocacy and educational role, it would link would-be housing providers with technical assistance and funders in the Partnership.

Single Parent Advocacy Network (SPAN). Several empowerment steps were involved:

1. The people who had indicated a concern about community support for single parents were invited to work on this issue. Four were single parents and two worked with single parents.

2. The issue was logged by the director of advocacy on behalf of the concerned group and taken to the Advocacy Committee. Prior to establishing a SAT, the group was advised to delimit the many issues faced by single parents outlined in the log and come back with a key problem on which a SAT could work.

3. The group recommended that single parents be "given a voice"—empowered to speak on their own issues. The Board approved a SAT to do this. Singles groups were asked to invite single parents to a meeting to identify their issues and begin to advocate on

those that were most pressing. Twenty single parents attending the meeting decided which were the most urgent issues.

4. Seven single parents volunteered to advocate on the issues processed by the group meeting. This led to the formation of the Single Parent Advocacy Network (SPAN). SPAN was made up of three men and four women who were single parents (5 divorced, 2 widowed), a board member who was involved in advocating on behalf of unmarried teen parents, a staff advocate who was a single parent and the director of advocacy.

5. The single parent members of SPAN decided that what they needed was a Single Parent Resource Center to provide crisis counseling, educational and recreational opportunities for themselves and their children, a library for both children and parents, and advocacy on long-term issues such as affordable day care, affordable housing, and legal issues faced during divorce.

6. The Board agreed to accept the Single Parent Resource Center (SPaRC) as a new program of the agency if SPaRC could find the funding. An advisory board composed mainly of single parents was set up and grant proposals were written; two grants were received and Phase I of SPaRC began in 1989 when a part-time counselor was hired to staff a telephone hot line and develop a library. Grant requests for a coordinator to develop a center in the downtown area were turned down. Finally, a new Family Service executive director who strongly supported SPaRC, convinced the Board that SPaRC should become a financed program of the agency and a full-time coordinator was hired.

The Importance of Structure

The structure outlined in the Flow Chart of Advocacy Issues requires further discussion.

The Log: This is where advocacy begins. The issue, based upon the system dysfunction and unmet needs or unmet rights is recorded. The log provides a beginning look at problems of people in the situation and in the system. The overall advocacy issue is outlined from case experience or other information. Then the problem analysis is begun: how many are hurting, how widespread is the problem, and to what degree are people affected? What legal or moral rights are not being met?

The log then looks at what would solve the problem. What change is needed? What would success look like from a professional viewpoint and from the viewpoint of those experiencing the problem? Will funds and/or volunteers be needed? Most important, who can make the changes that are needed? Who are the key decisionmakers? Within the target system, what are the forces of opposition and support?

Thus, the log briefly summarizes the problem, the possible solution, where change might occur, and who will be arrayed for and against the advocacy effort. It asks the same questions that will need more definitive study when the SAT meets.

Since the log is circulated for staff input and considered carefully by the Advocacy Committee, there is ample time for appraisal. Furthermore, the agency's mission, its advocacy goals, and the criteria for choosing issues provide the parameters within which the Committee considers or rejects issues and adopts them for continuing advocacy work (Taylor, 1987). For example, because of agency expertise in organizing coalitions, it was possible to envisage a coalition on homelessness and later a network of single parents regarding their concerns. No one else was taking responsibility for these and other urgent issues.

The role of the director of advocacy is to administer the program, enable staff, community people, and board members to work on issues, teach advocacy skills, and monitor (and often work on) SAT's to see that the study is done well and goals and objectives achieved. He/she compiles the annual report from SAT reports and analysis of the total advocacy process.

The *Advocacy Committee* is made up of four board members, four staff members (the executive director, the director of advocacy and two line staff), and four community members (representing various systems and client groups). A board member chairs the committee, providing liaison with the Board when he/she seeks permission to set up a SAT or reports on a SAT's study and action plan to gain its authorization to proceed. The two line staff members may (or may not) become staff advocates for a SAT.

The Board has a dual role: to sanction advocacy by authorizing Study Action Teams and, to participate in the advocacy work through representation on the Advocacy Committee and/or working on SATs. Note that the Board requires the Advocacy Committee to come back to it for approval of the SAT's action plan. Thus, the SAT is constantly accountable. In Lancaster, over half the board works on some aspect of advocacy in any given year, involved in the Advocacy Committee or on SATs. The Board assigns oversight and evaluation of the agency's advocacy work to the Advocacy Committee.

An *Advocacy Evaluation Subcommittee* evaluates the work set forth in the annual report prepared by the director of advocacy. The subcommittee adds its findings and recommendations to the Advocacy Report and sends it to the Advocacy Committee which in turn takes the full report to the Board.

The Study-Action Team. Each SAT must have a board member, a staff advocate, and community people (citizens, professionals with expertise and people who have experienced, or are experiencing the problem). (The latter can include clients, staff, board and/or individuals from the community.) All are invited to participate because of their concern, which ensures a high degree of motivation to work on the issue. The tasks of the SAT are to study the issue, develop an action plan, carry out the action, and submit a final report. In the event that it is unable to complete the work, a report is submitted as well. The staff advocate is the staff person assigned to a SAT by the director of advocacy to see that the SAT meets, is clear regarding its charge, and works with the SAT as a group to achieve its desired goal. He/she ensures that the SAT works within the agency's advocacy structure. Assignment of a staff member is made on the basis of interest, expertise, and/or responsibility within a department related to the issue. The staff advocate may be the director of advocacy, as was true in each of the advocacy efforts described here.

Why the Structure Works

1. There is total agency awareness and commitment before an issue is taken on. The Board commits financial support of the overall advocacy function and supports each SAT by its approval and its participation.

2. There is a clear understanding of the advocacy function in the agency and the role of each staff and board member. This is com-

municated when staff and board members join the agency. Periodic board-staff workshops are held to increase understanding and teach advocacy skills.

3. The fact that all members of the SAT come together as equals in problem solving and working to produce results, empowers them as an advocate group.

4. Study and action are inextricably linked. The expectation that something will be accomplished is explicit in the name of the committee — a study-action team. The structure ensures that this is the way it will happen by insisting on reporting back at the end of the study and action phases.

5. The structure assures accountability at every level: the executive director, director of professional services, line staff, Board. All involved feel a sense of control and an awareness that they will be clear about what the study-action team plans to do to deal with the issue. The fact that a board member is part of the study team no doubt reassures the Board. Similarly, the executive director can feel comfortable that a staff member is working closely with the volunteers. Community members feel a sense of stability in this structure as well. They know they are part of a process that has worked successfully on other community issues and that they are working with a respected agency whose board is behind them. Evidence of this comfort is shown by other community agencies readily allocating staff time to work on issues with Family Service.

6. The structure requires documentation at every point: the initial log, minutes of SAT meetings, reports to the Board, and the final report of the SAT, which becomes part of the annual advocacy report.

7. The structure mandates involvement of others in the community concerned with the issue. This is illustrated by the response of 80 community agencies, churches, and citizens to the invitation to understand who the homeless are, why they are homeless, and to work together to help the homeless and prevent homelessness. This community response was evident again at the annual meeting when people volunteered to work on community support for single parents. The agency's advocacy becomes the catalyst for people who are ready to work together in an organized way.

8. The structure involves people who are experiencing the prob-

lem (clients and others) wherever possible. They help other members of the SAT to be clear about the problem and feel it emotionally, not just intellectually. They increase awareness of those on the SAT who may be less familiar with social problems and what it means to live with them. At the same time, it can be therapeutic for the person who has struggled with the problem to be able to use his or her anger constructively to change or ameliorate a situation.

Reisch (1990) investigated the relationship between client advocacy and organizational structure in a study of more than 125 social welfare advocacy organizations in Maryland and Washington, D.C. Many of his findings confirm the validity of the Lancaster structure for effective advocacy. He found that effective advocacy organizations were more likely to have a formal organizational structure involving board and staff rather than informal communication between them. Also, they were "more likely to have established a structured goal-setting process . . . and to have maintained consistent goals over the past five years."

CONCLUSION

A structure that is consistently evaluated for its relevance to the agency's goals and objectives enables and empowers a growing advocacy program. It enables by clarifying and supporting viable issues; it empowers by accountability and a continuing track record of success. The latter also enables funding and continuation of advocacy work.

REFERENCES

Reisch, M. (1990). Organizational structure and client advocacy: Lessons from the 1980's. *Social Work 35*, 73-74.
Taylor, E. D. (1987). *From Issue to Action: An Advocacy Program Model.* Lancaster, PA: Family Service.

Mobilizing Women's Strengths
for Social Change:
The Group Connection

Alice M. Home

SUMMARY. Group work aims both at helping individuals cope with personal difficulties and at eliminating social problems through collective action. Women's groups have made a unique contribution to linking personal and social change through their explicit dual focus. This paper deals with the different ways women use groups to mobilize their strengths towards social change. It begins by explaining why women chose all-female groups as the primary tool for building both individual strengths and a social movement. Key features of different group types are presented, including those focused primarily on social change and those in which social action is a secondary goal. The paper ends with a discussion of obstacles to social change and some ways women's groups can overcome them.

Social work differs from other human service professions in its dual concern for personal and social change. The goal of helping individuals cope with the effects of social problems while simulta-

Alice M. Home, PhD, is Associate Professor, Ecole de service social, Université de Montréal, C.P. 6128, Succ. A, Montréal, H3C 3J7, Québec.

neously pressing for eliminating the causes of these problems is a thread which runs right through the history of social work. Group work exemplifies this characteristic most clearly through its trait of exteriority and through the existence of models covering the full spectrum of personal to social change groups (Papell & Rothman, 1983). In practice, however, the connection between "private troubles and public issues" has often been difficult to make (Schwartz, 1969). The Women's Movement has made a unique contribution to this linkage process through its explicit twin goals of building individuals' strengths and promoting social change in a group context. This paper deals with why and how women use different types of groups for social change purposes, as well as how they grapple with common difficulties.

WHY GROUPS FOR WOMEN ONLY?

Two unique features of the Women's Movement are of particular interest to group workers concerned about social change. The first is feminists' assertion that personal experience is at the very root of social/political change, while the second is the choice to use the small group as the primary tool for effecting change on all fronts. Many social movements have difficulty dealing with members' personal needs, because their male leaders often view personal change efforts as deflecting individuals' energies away from social action. Feminists distinguish between individual solutions which can weaken the struggle to change society and personal change which can strengthen individuals' capacity to engage in social action (Bunch, 1975).

This belief in the compatibility of personal and social change is one reason women were dissatisfied with mixed social change groups. As men assumed the leadership in both community work theory and practice, concerns of specific interest to women were dismissed as irrelevant "private matters." Issues such as child care and controlling violence towards women have been neglected by most mixed groups, and only recently have they begun to grapple with such matters as pensions for women who do not work outside the home. The tendency to treat women's concerns as "less important" is exemplified by the Canadian Native Rights Movement which has focused on the land claims issue, because of its importance in preserving Native culture and promoting self-sufficiency. Native women recognized the salience of this issue but were concerned about the loss of Indian status and rights by Native women who married white men. Children born of these marriages lost their status as well. This was clear-cut discrimination, as this law did not apply to Native men marrying white women. It was only after Native women organized an international campaign and a legal challenge that pressure was exerted on the federal government to change the law.

The lack of attention to issues in the "private sphere" is paralleled by a neglect of process and developmental aspects of group life. Community group work literature has finally begun to recognize the importance of dealing with personal needs and group process (Marcotte, 1986) as "the complete inattention to personal needs and interest . . . helped create and perpetuate an elitist model of organizing—one usually dominated by white males" (Burghardt, 1982, p. 13). Participation in social action can have secondary benefits such as increased self-esteem, feelings of mastery and empowerment, even if no particular effort is made to help members on a personal level (Levens, 1968; Rothman, 1974). However, failure to attend to members' needs for growth, change, support or services can be counter-productive in social change groups which need to recruit committed members (Lewis, 1983). Members need help in coping with the immediate effects of social problems while they engage in collective action to confront those problems (Poor People's Groups, 1973).

If mixed social change groups have reflected male styles and concerns, it is largely because these groups have been controlled by men. Although women are those most affected by poverty, old age, poor housing and inadequate services, they are often too isolated or too overwhelmed by sheer survival needs to become involved in social action. Many women (such as single parents) are unable to attend meetings scheduled in the evening as child care is rarely provided. The use of bureaucratic, hierarchical, formal structures by many mixed groups intimidates those women who do attend, making them hesitant to speak up. Perhaps most important, the norms and values of many mixed social change groups are in direct contradiction to those espoused by women. "Dominant models of community organizing stress 'macho' roles, tactics are often manipulative, power is construed as dominance, and democratic process and values may be sacrificed to achieve a desired end" (Weil, 1986, p. 206). Much community work theory is dichotomized into consensual models which collaborate with those in power and conflictual models. While women cannot support a power structure which oppresses them, they have been socialized to reject conflictual models emphasizing power struggles and confrontation. Even the vocabulary (strategy, tactic) is frightening to many women. Until recently, there were no distinct models, methods and structures suitable for women organizing social change efforts (Weil, 1986; Brandwein, 1981).

Women's lack of influence over the style of mixed social change groups does not stem from lack of involvement in these groups. Women have always been active in neighbourhood organizing and advocacy for oppressed groups, but their investment and leadership has often gone unrecognized (Côté, 1988). As their collaborative, enabling, facilitative orientation became subordinate to the directive, adversarial, controlling style adopted by many males, women's influence faded (Brandwein, 1981). Men became concentrated in high status intellectual tasks while women were relegated to supportive and technical functions (Lamoureux et al., 1984). This division of labour is typical of mixed groups of all types, which tend to select male leaders, even when women show more leadership ability (Denmark, 1977). Lack of confidence and group experience can prevent all but "superwomen," who are usually white and highly educated, from challenging men's leadership (Gallagher, 1977). In all-female groups, however, women are more assertive and androgynous, while being less defensive and stereotyped in their role behaviour (Toder, 1980; Aries, 1976; Mausert, 1979).

It is not surprising, therefore, that women decided to form their own all-female groups. What is unusual is the choice to make small groups the cornerstone of the Women's Movement. Early consciousness-raising (CR) groups were set up to help women "realize the full extent of their oppression and acquire a real stake in overcoming that oppression" (White & Goode, 1969, p. 56). The classical "CR" model encouraged personal sharing around themes to promote discovery of societal causes of women's personal problems, with a view to mobilizing members for social action. Despite the implicit goal of social change, however, many of these groups did not move beyond raising awareness and self-esteem (Home, 1981). Nevertheless, these combined goals groups continue to ensure the presence of a social analysis perspective. They have been helpful in promoting awareness of double oppression amongst minority, disabled, elderly and lesbian women.

As the Women's Movement grew, the use of groups became both more specialized and diversified. Although the priority placed on social change varied, the belief that the personal is political meant it was never completely absent. In therapy, support and self-help groups, social change is secondary to helping members deal with personal problems or develop new coping skills (Home, 1988), but social analysis is reflected in discussions about the impact on members of such issues as women's socialization (Gottlieb et al., 1983). These groups allow many women to develop the skills, confidence, autonomy and group experience which are needed for later participation in social change efforts. However, other women were impatient with the slow pace and dual focus of CR groups and formed all-female social change groups. The latter seek to bring about change not only in laws, policies and services affecting women, but also in community attitudes in order to convince the public of the salience of women's concerns. Services are seen as a way to draw attention to women's unmet needs while ensuring politics remain rooted in women's personal experiences. Many of these groups have formed collectives focused on mutual learning and power sharing in an effort to avoid male style and structures.

KEY FEATURES OF WOMEN'S SOCIAL CHANGE GROUPS

This section describes how the dual focus of women's groups and their informal, collective style influenced the goals, targets and structures of women's social change groups as well as their programmes and methods.

Goals, Issues and Targets

The integrated approach to change has allowed women's groups to shift priorities over time. In one Australian consciousness-raising group which had been meeting for several months, sharing experiences revealed that most members had had a rape or attempted rape episode. A discussion ensued about the pervasiveness of violence towards women and their reluctance to walk alone at night. After one member mentioned her previous involvement in a "Reclaim the Night" rally to draw attention to these issues, the group began to discuss the possibility of organizing a similar event locally. Eventually, the group decided to take this action, so the original consciousness-raising and personal change goals became subordinate to the social change goal.

This type of shift can also occur in personal change groups. A Quebec group was set up to reduce isolation and promote mutual helping among single mothers in a low-income community. The professional leader recognized the women's need for nurturing, as they had little support in their efforts to cope with their high-stress situation. Simultaneously, she expressed confidence in members' capacity to undertake social action. The group gradually spent less time discussing personal problems, and became involved in various social change projects. In an effort to reach others, they wrote a newsletter and a resource book for low-income mothers. They undertook action to change local school policies which discriminated against them. A major project was a play on the life situation of low-income single mothers, written and directed by the group. This humourous play, aimed at changing community attitudes toward single mothers, was performed in several cities. It had a profound impact on the group, on other single mothers and on the public. This group set up a Women's Center geared to the needs of women in its working class area. Throughout the life of this group there was a focus, rarely seen in mixed social change groups, on the members' double oppression as working-class women and on the need for simultaneous personal and collective action (Gingras, 1983).

The personal-political connection has had an impact on the choice of issues and targets for change. Early women's social change efforts sought to legitimize and act upon reproductive and child care arenas neglected by mixed groups. Groups espousing a radical feminist orientation focused on violence towards women, including rape and domestic violence. Other women concerned that the traditional sexual division of labour might be reproduced, sought change in the work world, through issues such as ending discrimination and on making working conditions more compatible with family needs (Wilson, 1977). During the 1980's, there was a gradual shift in the orientation of women's social change efforts from an ideological focus on naming and denouncing women's oppression to a service focus. This led to the development of innovative and diversified practices designed to meet women's needs in a variety of areas such as access to non-traditional work and shelters for battered women (Fournier & Guberman, 1989). Simultaneously, specific social change groups were formed in an effort to involve women excluded from the mainstream Women's Movement. In Quebec, for example, a collective of immigrant women is seeking change on issues affecting their members in the work world (unionization, language training, discrimination) and in the community (housing, health and social services, relationships with Quebec women). This trend towards more practical and diversified social change efforts has broadened support for the Women's Movement while causing some concern about both divisiveness and reduced radicalism (Fournier & Guberman, 1989).

Structures and Leadership

While women's groups vary in the extent to which social change is a primary or secondary goal, there is remarkable similarity in the ways in which these groups are structured. Most embody the feminist principle of power sharing through collective decision-making and shared leadership. At the same time, efforts are made to reduce dependency and to develop the leadership and organizational skills needed by women individually and collectively. Like other minority groups organized to promote interests of a specific population, these groups are low on structure, relying on mutual support and demand to influence members and orient group activity (Politser & Pattison, 1980).

A unique feature of women's groups is their explicit focus on reducing competition which often prevents women from valuing each other and from understanding and acting on their shared oppression (Gottlieb et al., 1983). One way this is done is through valuing and mobilizing the leadership potential of group members. Many self-help, social change and consciousness-raising groups avoid professional leadership to encourage members to use their own resources. As a women's self-help collective puts it: "Self-help groups can and do work without expert leadership. Women who share common experiences and who have struggled with a particular problem are well qualified to give one another support" (WCREC, 1985, p. 6). Some of these groups teach their members to help one another so that the trained women become resource-persons for new members (Glaser, 1976). Those groups which do have designated leaders ensure that they adopt a peripheral facilitator or resource-person role wherever possible, to avoid perpetuating women's dependency (Cardin & Home, 1983).

Skills and leadership sharing are especially important in collectives, an organizational form adopted by many women's groups offering services or working towards social change. Collectives' nonhierarchical structure means that no members hold special positions by virtue of their skills or status outside the group. Collectives reject the idea that experts with diplomas are the only people with skills. They do not believe certain (intellectual) tasks are more important than others. These principles mean all tasks are shared and everyone has the same right to speak and be heard as well as the same responsibility to make the group work (McKenzie, 1980). Members are responsible for recognizing and sharing their skills as well as for learning new ones, not only for ideological reasons but also to increase the political effectiveness of the group. When leadership and other skills are shared, the risk of dissolution if a leader leaves is greatly reduced. Finally, power sharing is ensured by the demanding process of consensual decision-making in which everyone discusses an issue until all members agree without duress (McKenzie, 1980).

Some collectives apply these principles to the letter, while others find it more practical to adapt them. One group which found that task sharing and consensual decision-making were not efficient developed a "shifting, horizontal leadership based on individual skills and time commitments" (Quest editorial staff, 1976, p. 41). Not everyone did identical tasks and some minor decisions were delegated, but rotating leadership in meetings and regular evaluations ensured the group could make changes before dissatisfaction built up. Another example of an adapted collective is a Canadian group which obtained a 3-year grant to improve services for mid-life women (Callahan, 1981). To avoid concentrating leadership, the paid coordinator role was rotated annually and part-time staff with specific skills were hired on short-term contracts. Women using the project's services were given the opportunity to develop leadership and participation skills through committee involvement. Some task rotation coupled with leadership development ensured permanent gains in skills extending beyond the life of the group (Callahan, 1981).

Methods: Program, Strategies and Tactics

Women's groups have developed some innovative ways of using program to move towards social change. Support, self-help and consciousness-raising groups use program which combines sharing personal experiences and information with discussion of societal causes of members' personal problems. Some of these groups use specific techniques to promote different kinds of change. The single mothers' group mentioned previously used structured exercises, sharing personal experiences and consciousness-raising techniques to promote both personal change and increased awareness of women's oppression (Gingras, 1983). A group of older women combined certain feminist counselling techniques (Russell, 1984) with consciousness-raising so that members received support while they discovered the specific oppression of elderly women (Hébert, 1985).

Leaders of a women's group in a Northern Ireland housing project made careful use of program to move members slowly towards social change. The group's goals included gaining self-confidence, learning about community institutions and taking social action. Although project initiators hoped the women would eventually take action, they helped them plan their own programme. Members were encouraged to confront visiting "experts" who knew little of their living conditions. Members gradually became active outside their traditional roles and developed an interest in areas other than child rearing. They formed a residents' committee to press for changes from the housing administration, did a radio program and met hospital authorities regarding that institution's treatment of women. The resource-persons gradually became less active as the group acquired skill and confidence. Despite the members' low self-esteem and an initial program emphasis on children's needs, this group was eventually able to take social action effectively (Lovett & MacKay, 1979).

Starting where a group is and using program suited to members' needs is the key to engaging hard-to-reach women. A social work student encouraged low income mothers in a new Australian housing project to get together for mutual support and collective action. The needs were clear to the worker, as there were no safe play areas on the busy street where the project was located and the women were lonely and isolated. However, as the women resisted all efforts to form a group, the idea of a resident's committee was abandoned and replaced by informal get togethers using recreation. Once the members began to enjoy being together, a picnic was arranged with women from a similar project who had succeeded in improving their living conditions. Later, the members visited the other project and began discussing action they might take. Had the worker not rethought the program, the group might never have come together. It is sometimes necessary to slow down social change efforts, to ensure members function well enough to work together (Hartford, 1971).

Once groups are ready to undertake social action, they need to develop appropriate strategies and tactics. A strategy is a long term, consciously planned action based on an assessment of the group's and the change target's strengths and weaknesses. Tactics are detailed methods of operationalizing a strategy. In deciding on strategies and tactics, groups need to consider both ideological and practical concerns. Choice of an appropriate strategy is often determined largely by a group's ideology. Groups which see unjust resource and power distribution as the source of members' problems tend to prefer a contest strategy while those believing that problems can be overcome by people learning to work together often choose a collaborative strategy (Gould, 1987). Radical and socialist women's groups tend to select a contest strategy, even though certain aspects are not congruent with feminist ideology (Weil, 1986). Ideological preferences should be tempered with realism, in that groups need to be aware of the practical advantages and drawbacks of each strategy. Groups need to assess their own competence, the likely resistance of the change target, the urgency of the situation, and possible consequences of using various strategies. Warren (1970) suggests assessing whether the principal parties have some basis for agreement. A collaborative strategy is advised when there is some common ground, whereas a campaign strategy can be used to persuade the other party when there is a disagreement on the perceived importance of the issue. Where the interests are irreconcilable, a contest strategy is indicated. Each strategy has its drawbacks. Collaboration can result in cooption or manipulation whereas contest strategies produce conflict and reprisals from the change target.

Successful women's social change groups often mix strategies to offset the disadvantages of each. When a woman was raped at knifepoint in a Canadian university residence, the authorities covered up the incident by announcing that as an "intruder" had been found in the residence, all students should be careful to lock their doors. Women who knew that the fault lay in an inadequate security system felt that only a contest strategy would be effective in changing the warden's attitude. After announcements were posted in an effort to destroy the cover-up, the warden and residents were invited to come to a meeting. Certain residents were prepared to ask him specific questions as to why the issue had been covered up and what security changes could be expected. A petition was circulated and the warden was told it would be sent to his superiors. This produced the desired rapid security changes as well as a lot of hostility from the warden. The women were careful to collaborate with him in setting up the new security measures, to minimize any long-term problems caused by the use of a contest strategy.

The demonstration project to improve services for mid-life women provides another example of the creative use of mixed strategies, in this case, collaborative and campaign strategies. Many women's groups get caught in the "compassion trap" of devoting all their energy and resources to providing services (Gould, 1987) which rarely survive the end of the initial funding period. Instead of responding directly to mid-life women's demands for courses, this group obtained a local institution's commitment to offer them on a permanent basis. The effective use of collaborative and campaign strategies allowed this group to avoid "zero sum games" which result in fear of change. The group created alliances with women in the target organizations, and remained cordial without backing down if change was resisted. They prepared a carefully written up survey of doctors' knowledge of mid-life women to obtain physicians' cooperation in changing their colleagues' attitudes (Callahan, 1981).

Groups need to look at how different tactics fit into a coherent but flexible strategy. They need to be spontaneous enough to take advantage of opportunities but systematic enough to ensure coherent planning (Henderson & Thomas, 1980). An Australian women against rape group had clearly articulated goals of pressing for legal change and raising public awareness about the pervasiveness of rape. The group used a combined campaign-contest strategy without making that choice explicit. Tactics were diversified and creative, including a phone-in survey of rape in marriage and a radio program on rape in war. The group's strength was its spontaneity which allowed it to take advantage of opportunities. It quickly organized a boycott of a violent pornographic film and participated in a proposed law reform after discussing the risk of cooption. However, the group was not adept at relating different tactics to each other or to overall strategy. This led to problems in recruiting committed members. Although new members were attracted to the group after each successful action, they soon left because of the apparent lack of direction. As a result, the group was dominated by a few educated middle class women who attended meetings regularly.

OBSTACLES TO SOCIAL CHANGE

Women's groups, formed partly as an alternative to mixed groups, have managed to avoid some problems typical of the latter. However, women's groups have encountered certain obstacles that are proving difficult to overcome. Recruitment and engagement are recurrent problems for all social change groups which must compete for members' scarce time and energy. Women's groups find recruitment especially difficult, because many potential members are already overloaded with double working days while others lack confidence in their ability to contribute to a group. In addition, the Women's Movement is, like many other social movements in their early stages, attracting mainly young, white, educated middle-class members who combine strong personal mastery with system blame (Rothman, 1974). Although feminist ideology emphasizes the universal nature of women's oppression, achieving solidarity and maturity as a social movement requires broadening the base of support and recognizing the diversity of women's needs.

In recent years, more minority and working class women have organized to ensure their interests are upheld. Reaching out to excluded women involves more than just inviting them to participate. Active efforts must be made to seek out leaders of different interest groups, to involve them in planning and to solicit their views on issues relevant to their communities. Aboriginal women's groups did not respond to an invitation to participate in an Australian rally/concert, presumably because outreach efforts were not thorough or persistent enough. A Quebec group planned a program featuring female artists to draw attention to women's accomplishments on the 50th anniversary of their obtaining the vote. Although the festival attracted many women who might otherwise not have been involved in the Women's Movement, an immigrant women's collective boycotted the event because its members were not consulted or involved in the planning.

Broadening the base of the Women's Movement is clearly a process which requires time, patience and sensitivity to cultural differences. Minority and immigrant women need to be involved in mainstream groups as well as organizing groups to promote their own interests. Two Australian women succeeded in setting up an immigrant women's group and involving them in speaking out in their own behalf. Before the women could attend meetings, however, the workers had to become accepted and trusted by their families who needed reassurance about the nature and goals of the group. Once in the group, there were linguistic and cultural barriers to overcome. Workers had to accept a slow pace of consciousness-raising because of the traditional role of women in many of the cultures represented in the group. Members needed much encouragement before they overcame socialization and cultural barriers against taking the assertive roles needed in social action. There is an expanding literature both on principles of cross-cultural group work (Glassman & Kates, 1989) and on working with specific cultural groups (Edwards & Edwards, 1984). This literature is useful in understanding certain difficulties, such as the Asian taboo on discussing personal problems with people who are not family members (Lee, Juan & Hom, 1984). However, many articles focus exclusively on therapy groups and few discuss specific obstacles in cross-cultural group work with women. The limited amount of relevant material is another reason for recruiting minority women to provide leadership on these issues.

Although more literature is available regarding working class women, they too need to be involved as members and planners/ leaders of groups. Persistence and a willingness to adapt program are vital to attracting and mobilizing working class women. Another key is offering services of immediate practical use to these women. A single mother on social assistance wanted to meet others in her situation for mutual help and collective action, but all her efforts failed. She finally started a clothing exchange which attracted many local women. As they got to know each other, they began exchanging baby-sitting services and discussing issues such as the lack of neighbourhood playgrounds.

Mobilizing women from diverse backgrounds implies awareness of cultural biases in feminist ideology and flexibility in its application. Feminist goals of consciousness-raising, building assertion and autonomy need to be applied cautiously because of taboos against questioning traditional sex-roles in certain racial and cultural groups (Home, 1988). Even in groups not coping with these taboos, there can be a strain between feminist ideology, sex-role socialization and practical demands of the situation. In some collectives, rigid adherence to norms of task sharing and non-recognition of skill differences can lead to poor use of human resources as well as wasted time (Leichardt Health Collective, 1976). One such collective insisted that a group worker spend her limited time doing the same individual crisis work as other members. The worker did some crisis work to show she accepted the principle of task sharing, while pointing out collective members' frustration at lack of time for outreach and consciousness-raising activities. Eventually, the collective agreed to let her organize groups for raising awareness and mobilizing women for social change.

The ideological stance that leaderless groups be used to encourage women's autonomy and leadership fails to take into account the extent of some women's socialization to passivity and dependency. Because many women are not ready for instant autonomy, "leaderless" groups can produce hidden, unacknowledged leaders who are often white, educated, middle class women (Bunch & Fisher, 1976). Many competent women hesitate to take on leadership, due to the insistence that all women can lead equally well coupled with the tendency to blame leaders for a group's mistakes (St. Joan, 1976). Groups can deal with this dilemma by providing some initial, time limited leadership. In one CR group, classical guidelines were adapted to ensure members had some capacity for autonomy while giving them the time to develop it. Group initiators recruited community women who had shown leadership potential while referring women in crisis to personal change groups. The resulting heterogeneous groups included women of different class and ethnic backgrounds at various levels in the consciousness-raising process. Heterogeneous CR groups are more likely to engage in social action (Home, 1981) but need more structure and leadership (Hartford, 1971). Accordingly, the workers negotiated a contract in which they provided some leadership for 8 weeks, after which the group could (and did) continue on a shared leadership basis. After the group disbanded, several members who had developed leadership skills set up other CR and social action groups.

It is not always easy for professionals to reconcile their training with the feminist focus on members' responsibility for leadership. Even when a worker succeeds in restricting her role to facilitating group development and helping group members mobilize their resources, she can have trouble judging when to intervene. The workers were acting as peripheral resource persons to the CR group planning the "Reclaim the Night" rally. They explained how to draft a press release and participated in preparing the rough draft to be put in final form by one of the members. This woman toned down the initial draft because it sounded too disjointed. Despite her reluctance to criticize this woman's initiative, one worker was concerned that the redrafted release would not get the media attention needed for the rally to succeed. As in many women's groups, the members said nothing as they feared hurting the woman. The worker decided that the risk of interfering with leadership was outweighed by the danger of the group's social action effort failing. She praised the woman for her work but expressed her concern, which freed other members to share their opinions and revise the press release.

While social change requires organizational, leadership and problem solving skills, members may be reluctant to take on certain "task" leadership roles. Successful groups need some members who can deal skillfully with the media, others who have negotiating skills and still others adept at political analysis, research or organizing. Women's groups need to assess what skills they possess collectively, applying the principles of task and skill sharing to ensure several members are skilled in each area. Members lacking confidence or skills can participate in training sessions inside or outside the group before sharing task responsibilities with more experienced members. Networking can be helpful in this process. The Australian women against rape group shared media skills with a CR group in exchange for the opportunity to circulate a petition at a rally organized by the latter.

Pace can be a problem for women's groups. They may delay action for lack of confidence or rush into premature action without adequate planning. Groups must assess their resources and skills, then choose a project they are capable of handling. It is better for a women's group to succeed in a small project than to fail in a large one or to delay trying for fear of failure. While the group is developing its skills by taking small actions, it needs to continue working on process issues. This is because social change groups need to achieve a level of autonomy and self-direction beyond that required of personal change groups. Groups must develop the trust, cohesion and commitment needed to cope with external threats, attempts at cooption and resistance from systems they are trying to change (Lewis, 1983).

Women's groups need to learn how to manage conflict within the group. As women have been socialized to avoid confrontation and feminist ideology rejects competition and conflict between women, many of these groups avoid facing the inevitable conflicts that arise (Hagen, 1983). Groups that do not go through the power and conflict stage (Henry, 1981) at the normal time must not assume that interpersonal conflicts will not happen. This stage often occurs later in women's groups which tend to deal first with intimacy issues. The late appearance of conflict can be misinterpreted as personal antagonism (Hagen 1983). In one research group, members assumed their common feminist perspective made discussion of process issues unnecessary. Dissatisfaction accumulated and erupted over power and task sharing, resulting in one member becoming the scapegoat and leaving the group. Failure to deal openly and quickly with early signs of conflict led to damaged self-esteem and reduced productivity. There are ways to prevent and manage conflict. Recognizing that opinion differences are normal, distinguishing between power and manipulation and doing group exercises (such as giving constructive feedback) can be helpful (Hagen, 1983). Establishing a clear contract and a norm of tolerating differences can produce a climate which encourages discussion of problems while they are still manageable.

The dual focus of many women's groups can lead to priority problems. Groups whose primary goal is social action may be uncertain about the amount of energy and resources to devote to services or action. Women's groups must be clear about their priorities and the reason for them. In CR and other combined goals groups, members may have different expectations regarding the priority to be accorded to personal or social change. Since these groups may change priorities, members need to be consulted periodically about the group's direction. When the CR group concentrated its energies on organizing the "Reclaim the Night" rally, there seemed to be consensus on the change in priorities. However, several members stopped coming to meetings, because they wished to continue sharing personal experiences but hesitated to speak up. Women are often at different stages in the consciousness-raising process (Guzell, 1977) with resulting variation in their readiness for social action. Just as groups must face conflict openly, they need to accept members' differing needs and continue discussing the implications of priority shifts until some agreement is reached.

A final issue confronting women's groups struggling for social change is the contradiction between the feminist focus on small autonomous groups and the need to come together in coalitions. Early feminist organizing tended to emphasize networking rather than forming strategic, multiorganizational groups. Coalitions do have risks, particularly because each group may bring hidden agendas or seek to dominate the others (Burghardt, 1982). When groups come together for short-term, specific events or issues, and when there is early discussion of the coalition's common ground, these problems can be minimized (Burghardt, 1982). In Quebec, women's groups seem to be adopting a strategy of short-term coalitions. Thirteen major groups came together to act on the question of secure funding for women's services and on a proposed reform of social assistance policy (Fournier & Guberman, 1989). The key issue appears to be whether acting in concert with others increases the chance of success without excessive risk to group autonomy.

CONCLUSION

This paper has discussed how women use groups to work for social change. Marginalized and unrecognized in mixed groups, women formed their own consciousness-raising and social change groups to deal with women's social action concerns without forgetting member's personal needs. These groups avoided many problems encountered by mixed groups, yet they struggle with issues of priorities, pacing, autonomy and leadership as well as the need to balance ideological and practical concerns. Women's groups bring a fresh perspective to social change endeavors, through their emphasis on power and skill sharing, participatory decision-making and building solidarity among all women. They are beginning to demonstrate how women of diverse political and ethnic backgrounds can come together to develop alternative services and press for social change on a range of issues (Weil, 1986). They have the potential not only to help women achieve integrated personal and social change, but also to influence the structure and style of mixed groups. A more participatory, process focused style would make mixed groups more appealing not only to women, but also to other minority populations who are hesitant to become involved in action for social change.

BIBLIOGRAPHY

Aries, E. (1976). Interaction patterns and themes of male, female and mixed groups. *Small Group behavior, 1* (1), 7-18.

Brandwein, R. (1981). Toward the feminization of community and organization practice. In Weich, A. & Vandiver, S. (1981). *Women, power and change*. Washington, D.C., NASW, 180-193.

Bunch, C. (1975). Self-definition and political survival. *Quest: A Feminist Quarterly, 1*, 2-6.

Bunch, C. & Fisher, B. (1976). What future for leadership? *Quest: A Feminist Quarterly, 2* (6), 2-13.

Burghardt, S. (1982). *Organizing for community action*. Sage Human Services Guide, Vol. 27, Beverly Hills, Sage.

Callahan, M. et al. (1981). *Prime time: A short-term project for long-term change*. Ottawa. National Health and Welfare.

Cardin, M. & Home, A. (1983). La pratique du service social avec les groupes de femmes. *Service Social, 32* (1-2), 170-185.

Côté, D. (1988). Les femmes en action communautaire: La genèse d'une présence silencieuse. *Breaking the Silence, 7* (2), 18-19.

Denmark, F. (1977). Styles of leadership. *Psychology of Women Quarterly, 2* (2), 99-113.

Edwards, E. & Edwards, M. (1984). Group work practice with American Indians. *Social Work with Groups, 7* (3), 7-21.

Fournier, D. & Guberman, N. (1989). Quelques défis pour le mouvement des femmes au Québec. *Revue Internationale d'Action Communautaire, 20/60*, 183-187.

Gallagher, A. (1977). Women and community work. In M. Mayo, *Women in the Community*. London: Routledge & Kegan Paul, 121-141.

Gingras, P. (1983). L'intervention auprès d'un groupe de femmes de classe populaire. *Service Social, 32* (1-2), 89-100.

Glaser, K. (1976). Women's self-help groups as an alternative to therapy. *Psychotherapy: Theory, practice and research, 13* (1), 77-81.

Glassman, U. & Kates, L. (1989). Group work method and ethnic-sensitive practice. *Proceedings: 11th Annual Symposium of the Association for the Advancement of Social Work with Groups*. Montreal 11th Symposium Coordinating Committee. 1059-1077.

Gottlieb, N., Burden, D., McCormick, R. & Nicarthy, G., (1983). The distinctive attributes of feminist groups, *Social Work with Groups, 6* (3-4), 81-93.

Gould, K. (1987). Life model versus conflict model: A feminist perspective. *Social Work, 32* (4), 346-351.

Guzell, M. (1977). Problems of personal change in women's studies courses in:

E. Rawlings, D. Carter & C. Thomas, *Psychotherapy for Women: Treatment Towards Equality*. Springfield (IL): Charles C Thomas, Publisher.

Hagen, B. (1983). Managing conflict in all-women groups. *Social Work with Groups, 6* (3-4), 95-104.

Hartford, M. (1971). *Groups in Social Work*. New York: Columbia University Press.

Hébert, L. (1985). Utilisation complémentaire de l'intervention féministe et du modèle de réciprocité dans un groupe de femmes ainées. Essai inédit. Québec. Université Laval.

Henderson, P. & Thomas, D. (1980). *Skills in Neighbourhood Work*. London: National Institute Social Services, Library no. 39, Allen & Unwin.

Henry, S. (1981). *Group skills in social work*. Itasca, Ill: Peacock.

Home, A. (1981). Towards a model of change in consciousness-raising groups. *Social Work with Groups, 4* (1-2), 155-168.

Home, A. (1988). Les groupes de femmes: Outils de changement et de développement. *Service Social, 37*, (1-2), 61-85.

Lamoureaux, H., Mayer, R. & Panet-Raymond, J. (1984). *L'intervention communautaire*. Montréal: Editions Albert Saint-Martin.

Lee, P., Juan, G. & Hom, A. (1984). Group work practice with Asian clients: A sociocultural approach. *Social Work with Groups, 7* (3), 37-48.

Leichardt Health Collective (1976). Structure, organizing and hierarchy in feminist collectives. *Scarlet Woman*, 4-7.

Levens, H. (1968). Organizational affiliation and powerlessness: A case study of the welfare poor. *Social Problems*. Toronto: MacMillan, 34-51.

Lewis, E. (1983). Le service social des groupes dans la vie communautaire: caractéristiques des groupes et rôle du travailleur social. *Service social, 32* (1-2), 32-49.

Lovett, T. & MacKay, L. (1979). Adult education and the working class: A case study. *Urban Review, 9*, (3), 193-200.

Marcotte, F. (1986). *L'action communautaire*. Montréal, Editions Albert Saint-Martin.

Mausert, R. (1979). The impact of women's groups on psychological androgyny. *Psychology of Women Quarterly, 3* (3), 241-247.

McKenzie, L. (1980). Small groups with WLM. *Melbourne Women's Liberation Newsletter*, 1-6.

National Council of Welfare (1973). *Poor People's Groups*. Smith Falls, Ontario.

Papell, C. & Rothman, B. (1983). Le modèle du courant central du service social des groupes en parallèle avec la psychothérapie et l'approche de groupe structurée. *Service social, 32* (1-2), 3-29.

Politser, P. & Pattison, E. (1980). Community groups: An empirical taxonomy for evaluation and intervention. In R. Price & P. Politiser. *Evaluation and Action in the Social Environment*. New York: Academic Press, 51-68.

Quest Editorial Staff (1976). Report to our readers. *Quest: A Feminist Quarterly, 2* (4), 41-44.

Rothman, J. (1974). *Planning and Organizing for Social Change*. New York & London: Columbia University Press.

Russell, M. (1984). *Skills in counselling women*. Springfield: Charles C Thomas, Publisher.

Schwartz, W. (1969). Private troubles and public issues: One Social work job or two? *The Social Work Forum*. New York: Columbia University Press.

St. Joan, J. (1976). Who was Rembrandt's mother? *Quest: A Feminist Quarterly*, 2 (4), 75-79.

Toder, N. (1980). The effect of the sexual composition of a group on discrimination against women and sex-role attitudes. *Psychology of Women Quarterly*, 5 (2), 292-310.

Warren, R. (1970). Types of purposive social change at the community level. *Truth, love and social change*. Chicago: Rand McNally, 7-31.

WCREC (1985). *A handbook for women starting groups*. Toronto. Women's Press.

Weil, M. (1986). Women, community and organizing. In Van Den Bergh, N. & Cooper, N. (Eds). *Feminist visions for social work*. Silver Spring, Maryland. N.A.S.W. 187-210.

White, P. & Goode, S. (1969). The small group in women's liberation. *Women: A Journal of Liberation*, 1, 56-57.

Wilson, E. (1977). Women in the community. In M. Mayo (Ed), *Women in the Community*. London: Routledge & Kegan Paul, 1-11.

The Use of the Group
and Group Work Techniques
in Resolving Interethnic Conflict

Alex J. Norman

SUMMARY. This article explores the area of interethnic conflict and, based on a case study involving a dialogue group of American Arabs and Jews, proposes a conflict resolution model that, combined with group process and group techniques, might be used to reduce tension and promote understanding among other ethnic groups in conflict.* The model was successfully used in Los Angeles to engage the disputants in social action during a five year period and shows promise of being employed in a new form of "intergroup work."

Sociodemographic changes in the United States, brought on by an influx of immigrant groups, are rekindling historical forms of interethnic conflict and creating new types of conflicts that promise to make the historical biracial confrontations familiar to us a thing of the past. In Los Angeles, Japanese American and Korean American high school students engage in skirmishes after viewing videos portraying Japanese as oppressors of Korean people, the result of

Alex J. Norman, DSW, ACSW, is Associate Professor at the UCLA School of Social Welfare, 405 Hilgard Avenue, Los Angeles, CA 90024-1452.

*A friend asked if I would help several of American Arabs and Jews start a discussion group, based on my prior involvement as a professional group facilitator (human relations and race relations). I agreed to be a volunteer facilitator and help them plan a discussion strategy. I became interested in the possibilities of participant observation techniques applied in a group setting and during the planning session agreed to facilitate the group. What I expected to be a short term volunteer effort extended to more than five years.

175

anger over the occupation of Korea by Japan. In New York and California, African Americans picket and boycott Korean merchants with claims of overcharging and racist practices. And in a California high school, Latino and African American students clash after African Americans walk out of a Cinco de Mayo celebration in retaliation for the Latinos walking out of a Black History presentation. The list can go on to include violence and death due to mistaken identities of a Chinese man beaten to death in Michigan when two white men mistook him for a Japanese and three Vietnamese assaulted in New York when a group of African Americans mistook them for Koreans.

These are but a few examples of daily occurrences across the United States. The situation is more critical however in the City of Los Angeles. Beneath that melting pot sits a "powder keg" of volatile social relationships in need of a mechanism that promotes understanding and reduces conflict. This paper proposes a model to engage ethnic and cultural groups experiencing conflict with each other in dialogue aimed at reducing intergroup tensions by using group process and group work techniques. A case study of American Arabs and Jews is used to demonstrate the model which combines social group work and conflict management techniques.

The nature of the conflict (tension between American Arabs and Jews brought on by events in the Middle East) and the composition of the group (subgroups of Arabs and Jews) required development of a model to address relevant issues. The author offers this approach as a mechanism for reducing conflict and increasing understanding between the descendants of the principals of the Middle East conflict, and one which can lead to social action. The model suggests an approach that can be used, albeit modified, to resolve interethnic concerns in a multiracial and multicultural society and promote cooperative arrangements.

BRIEF HISTORY OF THE DIALOGUE GROUP

The impetus for organizing the group came in 1983 from Sarah, a member of the Social Action Committee of a Jewish Temple active in peace and human relations movements, and from Alex Odeh, an official of the Arab American Anti-Discrimination Committee who was murdered a year or so later when a letter bomb exploded in his office. Events in the Middle East were having a polarizing effect on the attitudes and behaviors of American Arabs and Jews and, if left unchecked, the potential for violent conflict might become a reality. At two planning meetings attended by representatives of the Temple, the Social Action Committee and the Arab Anti-Discrimination Committee, those concerns and fears were discussed and the author suggested and explained the group process oriented nature of dialogue as a means of addressing those concerns.

The concern, that the politics of both Arab and Jewish organizations would discourage dialogue, was resolved by agreeing that this would be a grass roots effort. The fear, that public notice of talking to "the other side" might result in negative consequences, was handled by agreeing to keep a low profile and by not allowing "visitors" to group meetings. The concerns and fears were real. As late as 1988 there were fewer than seventy active groups engaged in dialogue on Middle East issues (Barkin, 1987; Bender, 1988). Recruitment of members was quietly conducted by a planning committee and "friends who could be trusted" to avoid group meetings being picketed or sabotaged, as had occurred in some previous attempts.

Although similar to the pregroup private phase described by Berne (1963) and Hartford (1971) in which the group or aggregate exists only in the minds of the organizer(s), this phase continued with the Dialogue Group well into the second year. Two reasons for this were the continued negative effects of Middle East conflicts on American attitudes and the death bombing of one of the Arab founders of the group. While certain group work principles applied, it would also be necessary to develop others as the process unfolded.

An original group of sixteen (13 Jews and 3 Arabs) began meeting in a Christian Church to resolve "turf issues" of both subgroups' reluctance to meet on the other's home ground (Temple, Mosque, home, etc.). The church provided a meeting ground for four monthly meetings during which time the membership dwindled to eight (5 Jews and 3 Arabs) for several reasons. Five Jews and 2 Arabs left the group when they could not vent their hostility at each other by "letting them know how wrong they were" and because they could not "set the history straight." Others wanted a more intellectual treatment of the subject and saw little to be accomplished by talking to each other. Even those who remained were uncomfortable with the process of the group and "felt" they should be doing something although they were not certain what.

The group worker/facilitator's role in the period of group formation was to help the group clarify its purposes and member roles within the vaguely defined objective of "getting to know each other." In an effort to increase the membership of Arabs the meeting shifted to an Arab Community Center, which caused the Jewish members to decrease to five but attracted two additional Arab members. The group of five Jews, three Arabs and a facilitator continued meeting at the Community Center. Afterwards, it met for two years at the home of one of the Arab members and almost three years at the home of one of the Jewish members until the group terminated.

During the six years of monthly meetings and social gatherings the group developed a statement of purpose. This was sent to other dialogue groups and distributed at local speaking engagements in high schools, colleges and Temples. The group sponsored and supported public meetings to promote peace in the Middle East. A team of an Arab and a Jew assisted groups wishing to organize. It maintained membership in national and local dialogue groups.

The high point was reached when the group agreed to two major media interviews. This was quickly followed by an actual meeting filmed for public television showing. By "going public" the visible support of Arab/Jewish dialogue gained acceptance as a means of settling disputes.

After the group's termination friendships remain, the closest of which are between an Arab, a Jew and the facilitator, who is African American. Recently the three had an opportunity to "tell our story" at a local Jewish Temple to members interested in forming a new group.

DEVELOPING THE MODEL

Although this was not a traditional situation for the social group worker it demanded a recognition of the democratic values for the common good, mutual participation (Coyle, 1947). It required interaction to solve a particular problem through an understanding of socioemotional needs (Bales, 1950). Its success depended on an acknowledgment of the interdependence of its members, not in a mutual aid sense (Northen, 1969), but of an ecological perspective (Toseland and Rivas, 1984). It required a willingness of group members to develop their capacity for cooperative living despite their differences (Wilson, 1976).

Unlike the traditional concern for the dual client — client group and the individual (Vinter, 1985), such group work is concerned with the total group, the subgroups based on ethnicity or culture, and the individuals within the group and subgroups. The tasks of "reduced conflict" and "increased understanding" were not clearly defined though they produced the same struggle between task and process described in Bales' work on group theory (1965).

The subgroup model of managing and/or resolving intergroup conflict was built on Walton's approach for managing international border disputes (1970) and Blake et al.'s workshop for confronting intergroup hostility between labor and management groups (1965). Walton's groups were not structured and lacked a substantive agenda while Blake et al. used a structured approach with a process for identifying agenda items and developing a consensus on priorities among them. Both focussed on moving from a win-lose (zero sum game) strategy to a win-win (cooperative) problem solving orientation by engaging the disputants in joint planning and collective action. Kitano (1974) calls this a *shared-coping approach*.

The role of the intervenor was to facilitate process with the group's time used as it decided in Walton's model. Blake et al. conceptualized a more active role with the consultant confronting, coaching, and challenging. Since both models were concerned with long-standing *underlying barriers* as the sources of tension, the author combined both roles into his interaction with the Arab/Jewish group. His emphasis was on facilitation of an open process of communication which might lead to understanding, not necessarily agreement. To this assertive facilitative role the author added the research methodology of *participant/observation* in order to ascertain the sociopolitical meaning of the activity and to capture a process in action from which to test the effectiveness of the model (Bruyn, 1966).

A major assumption underlying the approach was a belief that the historical complexity of the issues in the conflict precluded *right* or *wrong* answers. If there were perceived incompatibilities between group members they were to be managed, not resolved. This allowed for parties to agree to disagree on issues while promoting the understanding of some of the reasons for the disagreement. This may be applicable to other groups in conflict, where history serves as a barrier to progress in ethnic relations.

This approach recognizes that there are some situations which do not lend themselves to resolution, or the erasing of the origins of difference (Walton, 1969). It suggests that there are situations where success is measured by reducing the negative consequences of the conflict by increasing the understanding of why the conflict exists.

THE MODEL

The model has six steps shown below. Time is approximated. Although the steps are listed sequentially and appear linear, they often overlap and can be interactive.

Phase	Activity	Purpose	Time
1	Orientation	Information sharing, Setting ground rules	3 mos.
2	Group development of issues	Generating primary data for processing	3 mos.
3	Clarification of issues	Identifying common issues as a point for collaboration	contin.
4	Group diagnosis of relationships	Discussion/dialogue around roles and responsibilities	contin.
5	Action planning	Setting project goals and objectives for collective action	contin.
6	Monitoring/evaluation	Charting progress and planning next steps	contin.

Phase 1 – Orientation: The facilitator set the stage by informing the participants that the goal of the dialogue was to promote understanding between descendants of Arabs and Jews, and reduce the possibility of open conflict between them due to differences over peace negotiations between Israel and its Arab neighbors. He explained that he would be a part of the group as a member and apart from the group as a process consultant and observer, setting ground rules and keeping lines of communication open. Participants could discuss any issues related to Arab-Jewish conflict, agreeing to disagree on issues where there was an impasse. There were no preconceived ideas on where the group might go or what it might do but monthly meetings would be held to two hours. Thus, meetings were structured to change the win-lose relationship to a problem solving one which would *not include* specific grievances or personality disputes. Group sessions would not be used for counseling or therapy nor as opportunities to vent anger and frustration upon each other.

The facilitator's goal was to develop cohesion from the disparate interests of a group of professional middle class individuals. This was the *convening phase* in the context of Hartford's five phases of group development (1971). The period of group formation was characterized by a sharing of expectations, restlessness with the lack of a defined structure, withdrawal of members who did not feel the group met their needs, and a tendency to avoid disagreement and debate.

The facilitator was most active during this phase. At times it was necessary to stop a group member from verbally attacking another, so intense were the socioemotional issues. It was repeatedly necessary to clarify rules of conduct.

Phase 2 – Group Development: It was difficult to generate beginning issues for interaction through the fourth month when the total number participating had been reduced to eight, and the meeting place moved to an Arab Community Center. It was speculated that this move might increase Arab and reduce Jewish participation. A number of Jews withdrew, objecting to meet in an Arab facility. There was an increase in the number of Arabs attending, though it never rose above three.

When a Jewish member raised an historical issue, an Arab member would respond that his or her history books recorded it differently. The two different histories from the same events resulted in curiosity about how this could occur.

Sarah registered her surprise that the Arabs would resent Israel when " . . . they had taken that desert land and made it an oasis." Ahmed interrupted, pointing out that his family had lived for centuries in Gaza, "My father and forefathers farmed that land growing fruits and vegetables from which we fed the first Israeli occupation forces. I could get you some books which would help you really understand what happened there."

This led to a heated discussion and to a practice of exchanging books, newspaper articles, and community publications which provided issues for group discussion. It also produced the first "open fight" without fist shaking and finger pointing. It allowed the facilitator to point out the constructive consequences of heated exchanges, in that the group could move towards greater understanding though opposing preferences and antagonisms still persisted.

This also served to highlight the facilitator's role in the work group as dispute mediator. In such instances the facilitator must be even handed in his responses and behavior or lose not only credibility but the group. It raises the question of how effective a facilitator from one of the cultural groups can be, in light of the emotionalism of these issues.

Phase 3 – Clarification of Issues: This was the most difficult period. While both "sides" could agree that certain issues were valid (e.g., self-determination for Palestinians, a recognized State of Israel), and that trust levels were high in the group, each side held on to a basic mistrust of collective Jews and Arabs. Thus while the earlier phases were of approximately three months duration each, the remaining stages continuously overlapped each other. The facilitator intervened frequently as a process consultant, pointing out the tendency to win-lose behavior instead of a collaborative approach. He noted when each side was being heard or not heard by the other and that, while they trusted in the group, they were reluctant to trust outside the group.

The facilitator must be comfortable with ambiguity in the interchange of two different subgroups bound by ideology, history, and culture, attempting to find common cause in an environment which demands their cooperation.

A rallying point for all members was the feeling of agreement with Abba Eban's position on the Middle East peace question. It served to develop a sense of identity for the group.

This stage could be characterized as the *formation phase* in the group development process. The members become attached to each other, become important to each other, and attempt to influence the behavior and attitudes of each other (Berne, 1963; Hare, 1962; Hartford, 1971; Northen, 1969). For the first time group members had arrived at a consensus from points of extreme disagreement. This seemed to unleash, in quite an unusual way, affiliative interaction on stereotyping of Arabs and Jews, possibly as an attempt to show that the subgroups were more alike than different.

> Ahmed noted an increase in the stereotyping of Arabs as the ". . . bad guys with a big nose with a wart at the end." Sarah and Karen chimed in "That's exactly how they used to stereotype Jews." Mary noted how they were using the same words, "dirty Arab" now instead of "dirty Jew," and Rokiah added that since she was often mistaken for Mexican, she heard stereotypes involving both Arabs and Jews. She added ". . . and if we could just get together, nobody could top us." (You could almost hear her wishing they could get together.) Both Ahmed and Jihan said they were often mistaken for being Jewish yet both are Palestinian. We all agreed that they looked like they could be either. This brought a big laugh from everyone, almost like a release of tension.

Phase 4 – Group Diagnosis of Relationships: Group cohesion began to emerge during this period. Meetings had shifted to an Arab (Rokiah's) home. Solomon, who had attended with his wife Marilyn, revealed to the group that he had a terminal illness. The group listened to him, supported his efforts at rehabilitation, understood his need to make things "right" with the group, and, after his death, encouraged Marilyn to continue her association (which she declined to do). The facilitator helped the group deal with its loss as "our loss," and supported meeting socially between monthly meetings as a way of mourning. The death of a group member seemed to intensify the members' relationship to one another and to the world outside. Does trust in the group demand consensus? Should we recruit and accept new members? What will be our purpose beyond the quest for understanding each other? Over the next two or three meetings these questions were discussed and resolved.

Clearly the group had moved to the *group functioning and maintenance* phase in its history. The group could handle crises and began to reach out to help the community to understand the issues and what was at stake.

Phase 5 — Action Planning: During this time of planning for collective action another crisis occurred — the letter bomb murder of Alex M. Odeh, a founder of the group. The members were saddened, angered, and mournful over his untimely death and the failure to bring his murderer(s) to justice. Members were supportive of each other and used the outpouring of sympathy from the Arab and nonArab community to rededicate themselves to the cause of peace. Despite this low point in the group's history several action projects were undertaken to provide:

1. Technical assistance to other dialogue groups.
2. An Arab/Jew speaking team for Los Angeles high schools.
3. Group attendance at public lectures and films on peace.
4. Membership and participation in a National Coalition.
5. Sponsorship of public meetings on peace in the MidEast.

Phase 6 — Monitoring/Evaluation: By the fourth year of meeting, over 100 speaking engagements had been completed in City and County schools and on college and university campuses. More than 20 publicly sponsored gatherings were attended by group members. Members had been invited to testify before Human Relations Commissions. Two dialogue groups had been established on university campuses.

The facilitator used the accomplishments of the group to help bring about termination. The members did not want to accept that the attainment of its goals meant that the group could disband. It continued to meet regularly, supplemented by attendance at social gatherings, for another six months before working through the termination. Former members have remained friends and active in peace and human rights movements and, on occasion, see each other socially.

CONCLUSIONS

Analysis involving this small group of Arabs and Jews in dialogue suggests that the group, its process and group techniques, can be used to manage and resolve interethnic conflict.

Group work is rooted in the social action of the settlement movement, expanding the group work role beyond the agency to the community. In the course of another large immigration movement, group workers again have an opportunity to expand into the area of interethnic practice. The threat of violence to the welfare of children and families warrants such attention from social group workers.

The management of conflict model is useful because it avoids blame and encourages social action at the community level. The model of concerted action helps group members understand one another in time of conflict and, at the same time, provides service to the community through joint planning.

REFERENCES

Bales, R. F. *Interactional Process Analysis: A Method for the Study of Small Groups*. Cambridge, MA: Addison-Wesley, 1950.

Bales, R. F. Adaptive and Integrative Changes as Sources of Strain in Social Systems. In A. P. Hare, E. F. Borgatta and R. F. Bales (Eds). *Small Groups: Studies in Social Interaction*. New York: Alfred Knopf, 1965.

Barkin, R. M. "Participation in Arab/Jewish Dialogue in the United States," UCLA School of Social Welfare, Masters Thesis, 1987.

Bender, J. "A Look Into the Middle East Cousins Club of America Arab-Jewish Dialogue Group: A Piece of the Peace Movement," UCLA School of Social Welfare, Masters Thesis, 1988.

Berne, E. *The Structure and Dynamics of Organizations and Groups*, Philadelphia: J. B. Lippincott, 1963.

Blake, R. R. et al., "The Union-Management Intergroup Laboratory: Strategy for Resolving Intergroup Conflict," *Journal of Applied Behavioral Science*, Vol. 1, No. 1, 1965, pp 25-57.

Bruyn, S. T. *The Human Perspective in Sociology: The Methodology of Participant Observation*. Englewood Cliffs, NJ: Prentice-Hall, 1966.

Coyle, G. *Group Experience and Democratic Values*. New York: Women's Press, 1947.

Hare, A. P. *Handbook of Small Group Research*, New York: The Free Press, 1962.

Hartford, M. E. *Groups in Social Work*, New York: Columbia University Press, 1971.

Kitano, H. H. L. *Race Relations*, Englewood Cliffs, New Jersey: Prentice-Hall, Inc., 1974.

Northen, H. *Social Work with Groups*, New York: Columbia University Press, 1969.

Toseland, R. W. and R. F. Rivas. *An Introduction to Group Work Practice*. New York: MacMillan Publishers, 1984.

Vinter, R. D. The Essential Components of Social Group Work Practice. In M. Sundel, P. Glasser, R. Sarri and R. Vinter (Eds). *Individual Change Through Small Groups*. New York: The Free Press, 1985.

Walton, R. *Interpersonal Peacemaking: Confrontations and Third Party Consultation*. Reading, MA: Addison-Wesley Publishing Company, Inc., 1969.

Walton, R. "A Problem-Solving Workshop on Border Conflicts in Eastern Africa." *Journal of Applied Behavioral Science*, Vol. 6, No. 4, 1970, pp 453-496.

Wilson, G. From Practice to Theory: A Personalized History. In R. Roberts and H. Northen (Eds). *Theories of Social Work with Groups*. New York: Columbia University Press, 1976.

Action and Reflection in Work with a Group of Homeless People

Jerome Sachs

SUMMARY. The paper reviews work with a group of homeless men and women and explores contradictions which became manifest for the worker as he engaged clients who are economically and therefore socially and politically a part of an oppressed class. The work of Paulo Freire informs the discussion and illuminates practice principles toward a more radical approach to group work with poor, institutionally oppressed people. The paper also addresses clinical aspects of the group. The contention is that the historical split between social action and clinical work can be healed when work is focused at the psychosocial interface.

Social workers who see themselves as social activists have fewer professional and bureaucratic supports for their activities than they did at any time since the 1960's. Part of the reason is the systematic dismantling of the gains made during the War On Poverty in the last twenty years. Another, perhaps more important reason is the success social work has had in professionalizing, i.e, gaining licensure, increasing the opportunities for private practice, and becoming eligible for third party payments (Sachs, 1990).

Ironically, (Sachs, 1990) as social work professionalized it simultaneously began to give up its commitment to social activism, social justice and work with oppressed groups. As the profession and individual social workers gained status social work has become engaged, though not yet wedded, to the more conservative trends in the political economy (Cloward and Piven, 1976).

Despite this social work still remains one of the few professions

---

Jerome Sachs, DSW, is Assistant Professor, teaching Practice, Policy and HBSE at Smith College School for Social Work, Northampton, MA 01063.

187

with a rich history of social activism at both the clinical and policy level, and selectively continues to promote this tradition. Affordable housing and homelessness are two related issues in which the profession and individual workers continue the historic tradition of social action the work related to these issues that provides the backdrop for this paper. Attention will be directed to work still in progress with a group of homeless men and women (the group was established in November, 1989) in a rural town of 18,000 in New England.

The paper is organized around five phases or issues in the group's development.

1. The decision to work with the homeless.
2. The engagement process.
3. The first action.
4. Dealing with identification with the oppressor.
5. The current action.

This is a personal narrative and is therefore filled with distortions and omissions. It is, however, just these distortions which may reveal, for better and worse, the contradictions and ambivalences in values, beliefs, biases, countertransferences and theory assumptions (real and imagined), that precipitate a worker's action.

In so far as an outside observer, or workers themselves, can take account of the historic forces which make up his/her work, they can better understand the meanings of the worker's motivation and behavior (Schutz, 1967). For example, when I was studying for my Bar Mitzvah I read a story of how a great rabbi was struck with leprosy when he turned away from a calf being taken to slaughter. Years later, the story continued, the rabbi was cured when he fed milk to some orphaned kittens. Indeed my stock answer, when asked how I came to get involved in social and political issues is, "to avoid leprosy." As a trained analyst I recognize what must be a deep truth. The unconscious does not lie, however much it is filled with conflict, ambivalence, ambiguity and mystery. Both Freudians and Marxists understand the importance of consciousness raising. They are both aware of the freeing effect of understanding the motivations of one's actions through reflection.

. . . a revolution is achieved with neither verbalism nor activism, but rather with praxis, that is, with reflection and action directed at the structures to be transformed. The revolutionary effort to transform these structures radically cannot designate its leaders as its thinkers and the oppressed as mere doers (Freire, 1989, p. 120)

What Freire makes clear is that one of the structures that is often in great need of transformation is the mind and thinking of the leaders themselves. This is particularly important when one works with a group whose class interests, not to mention values, history, culture, race, gender and life style, are different than one's own and where one gains materially, however indirectly, from those differences, or when one's employment as a worker derives from the very existence of the social problem. Otherwise

the leaders [will] treat the oppressed as mere activists to be denied the opportunity of reflection and allowed merely the illusion of acting, whereas in fact they would continue to be manipulated — and in this case by the presumed foes of manipulation. (Freire, 1989, p. 120)

THE DECISION TO WORK WITH THE HOMELESS

Between 1988 and 1989 the Northeastern Housing Organization (NHO), a grass roots membership organization, made up of tenants, homeowners and housing advocates put forth a rent control by-law before the town council of Mapleton. The by-law was designed to control the 18-20 percent annual average rise in rent that had taken place in the town during the past five years. This was thought to be connected to the 32 percent increase in requests for emergency shelter over the previous year.

In 1989 the town council voted to put the rent control by-law up for a referendum. The selectboard and town council (both made up heavily of real estate interests), and local newspaper came out against the by-law. The campaign against the by-law was, at times, vicious. It included red baiting, harassing phone calls to women in leadership, misinformation and less than subtle intimidation of some tenants.

On the other hand, NHO consolidated its leadership in a six person steering committee, which included the author. The group's mailing list grew to over 150. Debates were held with landlords and realtors and consciousness about the need for affordable housing and homelessness was raised in the town. Though the by-law was defeated almost 2-1, it was the largest turnout in a bi-election in the town's history, and made NHO a force to be taken seriously.

After the election the core group of NHO licked its wounds, hired a new VISTA worker (the only paid staff), and rested. At the September meeting we shared summer experiences, assessed once again the gains and losses from the rent control campaign, and shared ideas about how we might work with and organize low income people.

The group did not have to look far. Some of our members and our new VISTA worker had themselves been homeless. In October the newspaper reported people living in tents in the woods while funds for a year round emergency shelter had been denied.

I had previous experience working with groups in an SRO in New York City. I had also been reading *Pedagogy of the Oppressed* by Paulo Freire and wondered whether his dialogical principles could be applied to work with a group of homeless people.

The dialogical theory of action does not involve a Subject, who dominates by virtue of conquest, and a dominated object. Instead there are Subjects who meet to name the world in order to transform it. If at a certain historical moment the oppressed . . . are unable to fulfill their vocation as Subjects, the posing of their very oppression as a problem (which always involves some sort of action) will help them achieve this vocation.

. . . in the dialogical task . . . leaders—in spite of their important, fundamental, and indispensable role—do not own the people and have no right to steer the people blindly toward their salvation. . . . Dialogue does not impose, does not manipulate, does not domesticate, does not "sloganize."

. . . cooperation leads dialogical Subjects to focus their attention on the reality which mediates them and which – posed as a problem – challenges them (1989, pp. 167-168).

By the end of the October meeting of the NHO there was a consensus to try and organize a group for homeless people. Three people from NHO would work together; Ellen a formerly homeless woman, Steve, a young paraprofessional who had previously been a VISTA in a food and clothing distribution program in town and I. In addition, Deb, our new VISTA worker, had recently been homeless and knew the network of homeless services.

Contradiction

I am no revolutionary. At best, and at times, I've been a radical, at worst, a liberal. I own my own home, am relatively privileged, and I know I would gain professionally from participating in the group. On the other hand, I'd be involved if there was no professional gain since I worry about getting leprosy. I also have a history of using my power and privilege to advocate and intervene on the side of social justice. Would I do so if I knew I wouldn't get leprosy?

Practice Principles

Social workers committed to reflecting on their actions do well to have other activists around. The more diverse the backgrounds of these activists the better. Everyone is kept honest by the different perspectives, and the possibility for "ego tripping" is kept at a minimum. In addition, the time commitment of the most disciplined volunteers, or even full time workers, is limited. It is essential to have backup. There is also a need to share feelings and ideas, ventilate frustrations, and be connected.

In our leadership group, for example, there was some initial deference to me as the initiator of the idea and the person with the most group leadership experience. The other two leaders, however, quickly began to play crucial roles in the process. For example, before the group began Ellen was quick to let me know that for all my book learning "social workers can really be terrible and don't understand the needs of homeless people . . . you have to be there," as she had been. At this formative stage Steve and Deb knew the social service system of the town and how to work it in a way that was beyond the knowledge, skill, or capacity of "the Doctor," the name Steve affectionately called me when he wanted to tweek me and bring me down to earth.

Clinical Work

It did not escape me that Ellen's anger had some transferential elements, i.e., was excessive and too repetitive (Freud, 1912). Though I often acknowledged the truth of many of her feelings about the destructive role of social workers with disenfranchised people, I also took the opportunity, as our relationship developed, to ask why she felt a need to deal with me as she did. Though I was a social worker and did make mistakes, I was also far from the "rotten workers" she described from her past.

On the other hand, transference always has a hook in reality. On reflection, I had treated her condescendingly. I thought it more important that I, rather than she, attend an important meeting. She was angry and talked about it with Steve who suggested she call me. She did and I apologized. She forgave me and has since been able to see me more as an individual than a "social worker."

THE ENGAGEMENT PROCESS

The place to find large groups of low income and homeless people in Mapleton is at the community meals program run in one of the local churches. I asked Deb, to make contact with the head of the meals program and determine if he would introduce us to homeless people. Happily, he agreed, and that week introduced us to two homeless men. The first question to us was "what do you want!" The question was anticipated. We explained who we were. We said we weren't sure we could be helpful but thought it worthwhile to see if we could. We hoped to meet with them, and talk about what their concerns were and what they wanted. The fact that Ellen could say she had been homeless was important, and gave us some credibility. They also felt good that we were all volunteers and didn't work for a social agency.

When we felt there was the beginning of a relationship, we asked whether they would be willing to meet with us after the meal the following week and if other homeless people they knew might be interested. They said "sure," but told us condescendingly that we really didn't understand. If the group ran late they'd get to their tent in the woods when it was too late. We quickly guaranteed transportation "home" to anyone who came to the group. Some of their skepticism disappeared. We then drove them, on a drizzly 35 degree night, to the edge of a secluded woods where they disappeared. I commented to my co-activists how strange it was to see them disappear. We all wondered how they would fare as the weather moved toward freezing conditions.

The following week three homeless men and two homeless women attended our meeting. Each told his/her story, and we were somewhat helpful in directing them to services that might help. We gave them names to contact at Legal Aid and the local community action office. We also gave them our phone numbers, and promised to follow up if there were any problems.

The group members also told us of the general needs of homeless people. We were learning. They were being helped, and the group agreed to meet again. By the third week we were twelve and by the fourth week fifteen.

Contradictions

When we took the men home to the woods the second week it was 30 degrees and snowing. After we dropped them off we talked about the contradictions of going home to our warm houses. We were also angry at some of the local politicians who talked about opening Town Hall for emergency shelter and then reneged. Though some emergency shelter money had been raised to carry the homeless to the summer, the shelter itself was not going to be opened for two weeks. The previous year a homeless person had frozen to death on the railroad tracks, and we were not willing to take homeless people into our own homes, however much each of us thought about doing so. It was easier to give money for food and be an advocate than to deal with what it would mean to have a relatively unknown homeless person share a roof with me, my wife and four year old child.

Practice Principles

In his discussion of cultural invasion Freire (1989) points out that

> . . . professionals (because of their very fear of freedom
> . . .) repeat the rigid patterns in which they were miseducated.
> This phenomenon, in addition to their class position, perhaps
> explains why so many professionals adhere to antidialogical
> action . . . Unconsciously, such persons retain the oppressor
> within themselves . . . they are almost unshakably convinced
> that it is their mission to "give" the [people] their knowledge
> and techniques. . . . Their programs of action (which might
> have been prescribed by any good theorist of oppressive
> action) include their own objectives, their own convictions,
> and their own preoccupations. They do not listen to the peo-
> ple. (p. 153)

Freire calls upon professionals to recognize how their behavior and actions are determined from above, face the contradictions in our relationships with oppressed people, overcome our fear of our own freedom, and engage in a dialogical relationship with the op- pressed. From this view some of the discussions about empowering people can be seen for what they are; another elitist, disrespectful, paternalistic, or maternalistic means of maintaining control. Some "empowerers" do not dialogue with the people, but rather proffer power from above, which, of course, can always be taken away.

An alternative view is that all people have power, and through the dialogical process begin to experience the freedom to use that power towards ending their own oppression and the oppression of others. Through this process both leaders and people become coop- erating Subjects in the historical process.

Clinical Work

Between group meetings I had the opportunity to encounter group members on the street and arranged to go with them to secure specific services. In the course of these extra group contacts we talked about "clinical" issues ranging from the need to get treatment for alcoholism, fears they had about having AIDS, ways in which they acted out their anger in self destructive ways when they were denied services, and ambivalences they had toward life and the world. They also began to share their hopefulness about the group, and the possibility that the group might have an effect.

In the group, members talked about writing a newsletter and other things they might try doing for themselves. This included inviting members of the Homeless Alliance, the planning organization for agencies working with the homeless, and the Organization of Houses of Worship to their group meeting. They also asked if they could participate in Homeless Alliance meetings. Homeless people were never consulted by the Homeless Alliance. Ellen, Steve, and I encouraged the group members' interest in asserting the power they had.

THE FIRST ACTION

The November monthly meeting of NHO took place after the second meeting with the homeless group. The three group leaders decided informally to raise the possibility of having an act of witness in front of the Town Hall; to open a town building NOW!, and not wait for the shelter to open. We polled NHO members informally and they agreed. We called the press. That night, in 20 degree weather, six of us stood, from 9-10 PM in front of Town Hall. We were freezing, angry and experienced the contradictions building. We knew that five to ten homeless men and women would be out in the cold the entire night, and that by 10:15 we would be warm.

Press coverage was good, but fallout from town officials and the local social service agencies, including members of the Homeless Alliance, was angry. "How could you do this knowing the shelter would soon be open," they said. We wondered why they didn't do it sooner when there were questions about the shelter opening at all. Despite this some organizations and individuals cheered us on privately, and less often in public. What everyone was sure of was that NHO had not disappeared after the rent control struggle.

The essential elements of witness which do not vary historically include: consistency between words and actions; bold-
ness which urges the witnesses to confront existence as a permanent risk; radicalization (not sectarianism); courage to love
(which far from being an accommodation to an unjust world,
is rather the transformation of that world on behalf of the increasing liberation of men [and women]); and faith in the people, since it is to them that the witness is made—although
witness to the people, because of their dialectical relationship
to the dominant elites, also affects the latter (who respond to
that witness in their customary way).

All authentic (that is, critical) witness involves the daring to
run risks, including the possibility that the leaders will not
always win the immediate adherence of the people. (Freire,
1989, p. 177)

Contradictions

There is a part of me that wants to be liked. I certainly do not like
to be attacked. The attack by would-be allies from the Homeless
Alliance was particularly disturbing. I knew we would have to work
with them in the future. I was also very new to this small town, and
worried about the fallout. On the other hand, I was also making
friends whom I liked and were supportive.

We were creating contradictions for the professional establishment. These contradictions would increase as they sent representatives to our group and as the homeless men and women became a
permanent part of the Homeless Alliance.

Practice Principles

Present talk of inadequate conditions is a cover for tolerance of
repression. For the revolutionary, conditions have always appeared right. What appears in retrospect as a preliminary state
or a premature situation was once for the revolutionary, a last
chance to change. A revolutionary is with the desperate people
for whom everything is on the line, not with those that have
time . . . Critical theory . . . rejects the kind of knowledge that
one can bank on. It confronts history with the possibility

which is always concretely visible within it . . . [Humanity] is not betrayed by the untimely attempts of the revolutionaries but by the timely attempts of the realists.
— Max Horkheimer — Quoted in Roderick (1986) p. 137

Activists in small towns need to understand that it's the next door neighbor or the folks around the corner whose interests they're opposing. In a city anonymity is possible. Small towns don't allow for it. My wife, for example, was greeted angrily by a merchant with "was that your husband!" This is another reason to work as a team, and not alone. It is also a good idea to find allies who are at least marginally a part of the "establishment" or have lived in town for three or four generations. "Outsider," "New Yorker," "Jew" were easy labels to put on me. Happily, it was one of the easier ones to wear since I feel comfortable and proud of the last two.

We were accused by other members of the Homeless Alliance of making a big mistake in this action. They voiced fears that it would threaten future funding and jeopardize current programs and that we needed to learn you could "get more with honey than vinegar." I worried whether this was true.

Clinical Work

The clinical work that was part of this action had to do with the exposure of my own deep rooted fears and rational and irrational paranoia. The rent control struggle exposed some of the individual and collective meanness that was present in the town. It scared me.

DEALING WITH IDENTIFICATION WITH THE OPPRESSOR: WORKING AT THE PSYCHOSOCIAL INTERFACE

In 1936 Anna Freud described the ego defense mechanism which she called, "identification with the aggressor." In the process of development children may, as a defense against anxiety connected with fear of outside aggressors, identify with the person of the aggressor, the aggression of the aggressor and/or the strength of the aggressor. By doing so children avoid the anxiety connected with a vulnerable and passive position. They become active, and at least in fantasy, may see themselves as strong and in control. In addition, they may externalize their own misgivings about themselves onto someone or something in the outside world, and vent their own aggression on that object (Freud, 1966).

In a similar manner, people who are oppressed may identify with their oppressors and attack others, who like themselves, are weak and vulnerable. It serves the oppressor well when people of oppressed classes and groups attack each other rather than join together to fight for social justice. Social workers as intermediaries between the ruling elite and the poor contribute to this when, for example, they are involved in making decisions about the "worthy" and "unworthy" poor.

Freire (1989) points out that leaders do well to "always mistrust the ambiguity of oppressed men [and women], mistrust the oppressor housed in [them] (p. 169)." In the homeless group it was often the case that members attacked one another, called each other "stupid," or defended the professional elite, saying such things as "you can't ask for any more," or "come on they [the 'unworthy homeless'] don't deserve anything, they're not even a part of our group." We also heard of the violence that took place between our group's members and other homeless people outside the group.

Parenthetically, it is worth noting that the group's only rule, one that has never been violated, is no violence. No one who was drunk, or angry, or "inappropriate" was ever asked to leave by the leadership. In fact the leadership encouraged people to stay even as other group members were shouting at them "to get the hell out."

Initially, the members of NHO took a clear position against the group member's oppressor within. The way we responded to their behavior could even be viewed as an attack on the members themselves. For example, we indicated that they were acting and talking just like the workers in the agencies which had denied them services. Recently we posed the question; "what does it mean and how is it that we so often experience you as attacking one another?" The discussion that took place raised both political and psychological consciousness as they recognized how they acted out their frustrations and anger on each other and themselves rather than directing it at those who deserved it. They began to recognize that their energies could be used collectively to help one another. It was a major breakthrough which was to have important implications in the next phase of the group process.

Contradictions

Were we acting as oppressors when we took a stand against the group member's oppressor within? The question suggests the answer and our reflection, which led to posing a dialogical problem, certainly led to better results. On the other hand, and this may be a rationalization, it allowed a number of group members to disagree with each other and the leadership. We all learned we could continue to work together while respectfully, though heatedly, disagreeing.

Practice Principles

Leaders must also be aware of their own and the oppressed's ambiguous relationship to oppression. It is only by posing this ambiguity itself as a dialogical problem that it becomes possible to develop the communion and cooperation that Freire talks about.

> In dialogical theory, at no stage can the revolutionary forgo communion with the people. Communion in turn elicits cooperation, which brings leaders and people to the fusion, described by [Che] Guevera. This fusion can exist only if revolutionary action is really human, empathic, loving, communicative and humble, in order to be liberating. (1989 p. 171)

It is at this level of work that the false dichotomy between clinical work and social action disappears and is seen for what it is; a way to maintain privilege and split the profession from itself and the people with whom its progressive wing has historically worked.

THE CURRENT ACTION

The town's emergency shelter was scheduled to close May 1. In previous years residents of the shelter would again move to the woods, go to another town that had a year round shelter, sleep in doorways or a dumpster, or try to move in with a sympathetic relative or friend.

This year the group asked that I pose the issue of where they would go to the Homeless Alliance and suggest that, if a town building or other suitable dwelling was not found, they were prepared to set up tents and sleep on the town common. There was great resistance from the town's politicians and from the right wing of the social service community which called an "emergency meeting" to berate me personally. They neglected to invite the men and women of the homeless group even though they said they had when they called me the night before for an 8 AM meeting the next day. The "tent in" was, however, scaled down to a noon to 9 PM vigil after money "magically" appeared for motels for any homeless person who needed it that week.

In the course of the week the town fathers agreed to use the Town Hall as shelter from 8 PM to 7 AM until one of the local agencies could get a back room in shape to house homeless people on a more permanent basis. The 9 hour vigil was successful. It was run almost completely by the group members. The continued threat of a tent-in no doubt had something to do with finding money and space to house the homeless.

Contradictions

At this stage of the group there was a true fusion between the leadership and the group's members. Leadership was shared according to known abilities and interests. There was much mutual support. I felt truly communed with when homeless men and women and my co-activists defended me at the Homeless Alliance meeting which followed the "emergency meeting." As one of the homeless men said to me, recalling Horkheimer, "sure you make mistakes, its because you bother doing something."

Contradictions, which did exist, were experienced by members of the Homeless Alliance who had resisted the action. Their psychological stress was painful to watch, and some of us tried to help them come to terms with it. I suggested that it was clearly painful for them when they wanted to help and, at the same time, maintain their good relations with those in town who opposed homeless people taking control over their lives.

Fortunately, there was the happy coincidence of a new member in the Homeless Alliance. Ed was a pacifist. He was also an ideological ally of both NHO and the homeless. We suggested he assume the role of the stranger (Simmel, 1950) and chair the Homeless Alliance meetings at this tumultuous time.

Practice Principles

The dual principles of action and reflection are worth reiterating. The ability to share and relinquish leadership to the people is essential. Unification of the homeless with other oppressed people takes place through praxis.

> In order for the oppressed to unite, they must first cut the umbilical cord and myth which binds them to the world of oppression. . . . Since the unity of the oppressed involves solidarity among them, regardless of their exact status, this unity unquestionably requires class consciousness. (Freire, 1989 pp. 174-175)

As noted, it is also useful to have an ally who can take a mediating position when necessary.

Clinical Work

The recognition and collective constructive use of their power had both a therapeutic and, I believe, immunizing effect on every member of the group and other homeless and poor people who joined the vigil during its nine hours. As one usually deeply despairing and depressed man in the group said to me, "I really feel good about being involved." Another woman who we hadn't seen in the group for some time said, "you really did it." It was good for the leaders too. Women and men don't have to identify with the aggressor or the oppressor when they affirm their own self worth and the worth of others.

CONCLUSION AND A FINAL CONTRADICTION

As of this writing (June, 1990) the Town Hall is open. Volunteers, including some formerly homeless men from the group, are providing security. Some of the churches have mobilized to help with food, clothing and other needs beyond what they had done in the past.

But eight new homeless people have emerged. More will arrive and as Ed, the pacifist, pointed out to me when I was feeling overly optimistic about the gains we had made, "at best it's still shit." On the other hand, no one in the group is sleeping in the woods or a dumpster. The work that was done will be a base to build on for the future.

REFERENCES

Cloward, R.A. and Piven, F.F. (1976). Note toward a radical social work. In F. Bailey and M. Brake (Eds.) *Radical social work*. pp. vii-xlvii. New York: Pantheon.

Freud, A. (1966). *The ego and the mechanisms of defense*. New York: International Universities Press.

Freud, S. (1912). *The dynamics of transference*. In Freud, S. *Therapy and technique*. Philip Rieff (Ed.). New York: Crowell-Collier.

Freire, P. (1989). *Pedagogy of the oppressed*. New York: Continuum.

Roderick, R. (1986). *Habermas and the foundations of critical theory*. New York: St. Martin's Press.

Schutz, A. (1967). *Phenomenology and the social world*. Evanston: Northwestern University Press.

Sachs, J. (1990). Professionalism, licensure, private practice and the decline of social commitment. *BCR Reports: Newsletter of the Bertha Capen Reynolds Society, 2*, 1-5.

Simmel, G. (1950). *The Sociology of George Simmel*. New York: The Free Press.

The Relevance of Stages
of Group Development Theory
to Community Organization Practice

Jacqueline B. Mondros
Toby Berman-Rossi

SUMMARY. Community organizers are concerned with the development of a large and invested group of participants. A working knowledge about how groups come together and evolve is indispensable if organizers are skillfully to develop relations among members, create a mutual aid system, and handle the initial authority theme. In this paper, a community organizer's attempts to build a group are presented and analyzed according to stages of group development theory.

As community organizers go about the business of acquiring influence to induce change on specified issues, they need simultaneously to be concerned about building groups that are large, invested, and readied for work.[1] Having such a working group enables the organization to be in an ongoing state of readiness to pursue new issues and negotiate agreements with external systems. Without such a group, organizers are forced to recreate an organization as each new organizing effort is undertaken.

Since organizers work to develop such groups, they should be deliberately attentive to how groups develop, function, and are sus-

---

Jacqueline B. Mondros, DSW, and Toby Berman-Rossi, DSW, are affiliated with the Columbia University School of Social Work, 622 W. 113th St., New York City, NY 10025.
The authors wish to thank Irving Miller for his generous editorial assistance, and NM for providing the illustrative material on which our discussion of MITE is based.

203

tained. Actually, the organizer's interest in achieving valued outcomes often overshadows and diverts attention from the relationship between group development and organizational achievements.[2]

Organizers perform four primary activities in the initial stages of an organizing effort: (1) tuning in to and preparing for the recruitment of potential members and the ensuing group meetings; (2) actually recruiting people; (3) engaging new people and the group in the beginning phase of work; and (4) sustaining the group as issues of ownership arise.[3]

There are numerous pitfalls in each activity, and organizers invite trouble for themselves if they don't attend to how and why people join groups, the meaning of group experience for individuals, and matters of group process during these beginning efforts.[4] Organizers incorrectly assume that people join solely out of interest in issues and prepare themselves to discuss only the issues and desired ends. Consequently they may fail to detect cues about the secondary expressive concerns of members. In group meetings, particularly initial ones, organizers may wrongly assume only instrumental matters are important and in order.

When recruiting, organizers often believe that the people with whom they have had initial contact will enthusiastically join and participate. Because they impute universal zeal they place unrealistic demands upon them. New recruits may shrink from this overly eager approach. When people don't readily join, organizers assume disinterest at best; at worst, they decry their lack of activism. The organizer's disdain may be communicated to potential members and further alienate them. Such presumptions by the organizer can cut the embryonic organization off at its conception.

Organizers find many ways to explain why new recruits don't return to a newly formed group. They frequently say that people are too busy, i.e., they believe the standard excuses, lose interest, or, more pejoratively, see their commitments as shallow. Such assumptions may intensify a tendency to make greater demands on remaining members. Then, membership fall off deprives the group of the infusion of the ideas that new members bring. New recruits sitting on the sidelines have no incentive to remain involved.

Organizers tend to assume that a group once formed should continue to operate harmoniously. They view the emergence of conflict, difference, and vying for power as threatening the work of the group and possibly their own authority. This belief entices the organizer to avoid conflict by controlling group process. Such control can produce the very behavior the organizer wishes to avoid.

When organizers succumb to any or all of these pitfalls, potential members may not join, the group may not really develop, or may dissolve prematurely. Moreover, the group may become totally controlled by the organizer's own preferred outcomes and methods for achieving them.

Group workers are educated to see ambivalence and concerns about power and control as normative aspects of group participation and group process. It would be helpful if organizers develop similar understanding and comfort with the idea that such behaviors are to be expected. They will, in effect, have more realistic expectations of newcomers and new groups. As a consequence their practice may be more attuned to what happens in the beginning phase of group development. The pay-off is fewer problems, and a more mature group, better able to do its current and future work.[5]

In the pages which follow we will describe the four primary tasks the organizer performs in the early stages of an organizing effort. We will show the pertinence of stages of group development literature to the special features of community organization practice[6] and will illustrate the ways in which this literature informs community organization practice.

Although there are many common elements in group work and community organization practice, there are certain distinctions. These distinctions influence how stages of group development literature informs community organization practice. Organizers have two common objectives when they come into a community: to empower people and to redistribute existing power.[7] To pursue the first objective, the organizer validates people's perception of shared problems, offers and encourages hope that something can be done about it,[8] and proffers technical assistance in studying issues and designing strategies to achieve their goals. Helping people do for themselves is the primary aim. The organizer is an enabler, teacher, and resource provider and is not a formal leader who acts on behalf of others. The second objective, i.e., the redistribution of power, can be pursued as people learn to act in their own behalf and experience a sense of competence. Embued with such strength they begin to see a need for an organization, continuously and vigilantly, to represent their common interests. The organizer then helps them to establish a structured and disciplined organization in which they all are mutually accountable to each other. The organization then can negotiate with powerholders on a firmer footing and in an ongoing way.

When organizers come into a community this vision of what can or might be is largely in their imagination. There is a large distance between the organizer's vision and how people feel about the possibility of change. Commonly, people will not readily make an effort to initiate change simply because their lives are oppressive. They view community problems as overwhelming and immutable, resign themselves to live with them, and are wary of promoting social change. Becoming involved in an organizing effort forces people to begin to question the legitimacy of entrenched and traditional power. They begin to redefine their own deeply held notions about who they are, their role in their community, and the degree of influence they might have. As a result, people will initially be skeptical about, if not daunted by, the prospect of making significant changes in their community.

Working in even the most homogeneous communities, community organizers inevitably discover and rediscover that people are as much unlike as they are like each other. There are the obvious racial, ethnic, age, and class interests which divide people and make it difficult to achieve consensus. People also differ by the degree of influence they have in the community's power structure, and therefore have different allegiances to it. While generally people do not want to antagonize public officials, those with political entree will be least disposed to rock the boat. They will tend to resolutely guard their own prerogatives. Thus, some will be assertive and others cautious on the subject of change.

CASE ILLUSTRATION

The following material is selected from "Midburg Interfaith Training and Empowerment" (MITE) a community group in the small northeastern city of Midburg. It represents many of the patterns and problems typical of community organizations in their early stage of development and also has some interesting distinctive features.

Midburg was a declining small city, fraught with crime, poor city services, a failing school system, an expensive yet deteriorating housing stock and sharp racial and economic divisions. Many residents were disillusioned and felt very pessimistic about the City's future. While divisions among people are apparent in the beginning stages of most organizing efforts, Midburg was particularly marked by such tension. The City has had a long history of racial and economic polarization and fanning the fires of fear has not been beneath most of the city's politicians. As a city of 200,000, it is small enough to give the impression that influence is possible. In fact, access to power is not equal. The City is heavily Catholic, and priests, particularly those from white middle class parishes, have had easier access to the political power structure and have been able to negotiate preferred arrangements for themselves and their parishes.

Concern about the problems in Midburg led a group of Catholic clergy to raise money to hire a community organizer with the responsibility and sanction to organize their parishes. There were, of course, differences among them. Priests from white, middle class parishes entered into agreements cautiously, careful to protect the autonomy of their churches and wary about upsetting their relationships with public officials. Those from the poor Hispanic sections eagerly supported the idea of an organization which would assertively pursue the serious problems of their parishioners.

In 1986 an organizer was hired to bring residents together to begin to identify and work on City problems. Initial organizing efforts were successful. Local issues were identified, developed, and successfully resolved. In 1987, a loose and flexible organization of area churches and synagogues was formed. It was disciplined enough for further action, and open enough to allow new people to join. Four officers were elected and agreement was reached to form MITE. The name was chosen to suggest its potential for power building.

The organizer reached out to Midburg residents to help them identify common issues and to lend his expertise so they could formulate successful strategies. Groups, under the auspice of MITE, achieved success on many issues, including establishment of a co-op conversion fund law, assignment of a Police Task Force to public housing, publication of the first City Information Handbook, and development of the first comprehensive plan for low-income, middle income, and luxury housing.

Despite these successes, serious differences threatened a fragile consensus as well as the organization itself. There were frequent debates about who should join, what issues should be undertaken, and how assertively the organization should pursue its interests.

In the spring of 1990, MITE members met with the Catholic pastors ostensibly to discuss the issues they later felt the organization should pursue. Additionally, they sought to involve those priests who had kept their distance. One of these, Father C., told them he was interested in doing something to get a new library built in Midburg, an issue which like much else in the City, had a long and ambiguous history.

In the 1970s, the State purchased and demolished the old library, widening the road downtown in order to attract business. At the time of the purchase, the City Council promised to build a new library on the same site. Instead, the library was "temporarily" moved to a vacant department store in a dilapidated downtown section. Twenty years later, the cost of a new library had more than doubled. It has not been built because of "fiscal constraints" though every fiscal year the City budget included funds for building the library. In sum, the library building was a cause anyone could warm to, including Father C., the cautious priest. Equally important, it was a problem that could be solved if people worked together to apply pressure.

How knowledge of stages of group development informed the organizer's practice as he recruited for and worked with a group interested in a new City library can now be described and analyzed.

Tuning In and Recruiting New Members

The organizer's initial contact with potential group members can determine whether or not they become involved. Knowledge of how groups develop can inform the recruiting efforts of organizers.

Even though stages of group development literature concerns itself with already formed groups and does not explicitly deal with recruiting, inferences about outreach can be drawn. Understanding the range of what is often experienced in initial group meetings guides the organizer (and others who work with formed groups) on how to go about inviting potential members into the group. What organizers tell individuals about the group and how they prepare them for the experience contribute to an individual's decision to participate and/or remain in the group. In addition to the lure of the issue, a prospective recruit's decision will be influenced by the experience with the organizer. For this experience to be positive the organizer will have to tune into and be responsive to possible ambivalence, reluctance, or other concerns which inhibit joining. An example will illustrate.

Preparing to Recruit for the Library Committee: As I tuned into this meeting with Kate, my hunch was that as a literacy volunteer, Kate would have a natural interest in a library. Yet, as a former teacher she was likely to have a penchant for order and structure and might be anxious in the beginning when norms of conduct and a structure for work had yet to be developed. I set out to test Kate's interest and whether there was sufficient common ground to warrant my encouraging her attendance. I wanted her to be clear about why we were meeting and what involvement with the Library Committee might entail. While we agreed to meet to talk about the library, I knew Kate might still be cautious and tentative about getting involved. Wanting a library was not the same as becoming involved in getting one. I knew that I would need to be responsive to any subtle hesitancy, for in that hesitancy might be found Kate's reasons for remaining on the sidelines.

Recruiting Kate: From the beginning, we reviewed our agreement about why we were meeting. We made explicit our shared interest in a new library and acknowledged that we were meeting to think together about the library. I asked Kate what she thought about the library. I shared my view and remarked on how similar our views were. Kate spoke little about how she felt working in a "temporary" library for 10 years, and where all agreed that the working conditions were unpleasant. I asked Kate what she remembered about the old library, hoping that I could arouse some emotion. At this point Kate came alive. She reminisced about getting her library card at the old library and about the old neighborhood. There was sadness in her voice as she spoke about how bad things are now. I told Kate she had given me a vivid historical picture and helped me understand better why the library is so important to people.

We were quiet for a moment. Slowly Kate said that it is difficult to do anything. Sensing her hopelessness, I said I believed that it was important for people to stand together to do anything at all and that there is a need for people to act and to propose solutions rather than just to react. Still unconvinced that she could have a hand in solving the problem, Kate said she thought the library director would be doing something to get the City to fulfill its 20 year promise. We talked about how difficult it would be for the director, as a salaried City employee, to act and how an outside group would have greater license. She understood. I wondered if she would like to interview some people with me to find out where the building of the library stood now. I proposed this because we could continue developing our relationship as we gathered information. I intuited, however, she worried that these interviews would be complicated and she would not be up to the task. Kate reluctantly agreed. Together we formulated the questions we would ask. I provided information so Kate could come to these interviews with greater confidence.

The organizer's work with Kate was guided by his knowledge that many people are reluctant to involve themselves in groups. While a less skilled organizer might drive home the issue by talking about action, this organizer understood that Kate's initial involvement was tentative. Recognizing Kate's hesitancy, he encouraged her to regain a sense of her investment, to confirm it, to contrast it with the past, and to reconfirm her desires for the present. Sensing her reluctance, he drew out her fears, her ambivalence, and myths which inhibited action. Not making demands too early allowed

Kate to invest at her own more comfortable pace. Finally, he invited Kate to become active. He structured an activity, provided information, and worked with her to increase her sense of competence. Throughout, he shared his knowledge and affirmed Kate's expertise as a community resident so they could work as mutual "experts."

His actions were designed to increase Kate's sense of competence and to equalize their power in the relationship. In so doing he enhanced her willingness to act outside and within the group. Once in the group, Kate's increased knowledge and greater self-confidence would strengthen the group as a whole.

INITIAL STAGES OF GROUP DEVELOPMENT

Stage I: Pre-Affiliation: Engaging Individuals and the Group in the Initial Stage of Work

As organizers bring new recruits to an initial meeting, they face new challenges. They must recognize the uncertainty and wariness which accompany group beginnings. Strong commitment to the cause of the group may be necessary, but it is not necessarily sufficient to keep people invested in the enterprise. In Stage I, Pre-Affiliation,[9] people are a collection of separate individuals, with a potentially wide range of views and some hesitancy to communicate too directly. This state establishes the first task, developing a shared definition of the work to be done. Lacking formal authority, community organizers cannot use their influence directly but must engage the members in discussion of purpose, goals, and structure for work as a basis for their groups to become self-directing with a culture which supports work, direct communication, and mutuality.

Stage II: Power and Control

Sustaining the Group as Issues of Ownership Arise

Once it has agreed on a contract for work, the group has two primary tasks: (1) to develop into a mutual aid system from which trust, rules of behavior, norms, and a structure for work may be established, and (2) to determine to whom the group belongs.

Group members usually become concerned with asserting themselves, and with who "owns" the group. Challenges, self-assertion, and active disagreement are common. In this early stage members are preoccupied with power and control issues, i.e., their relationship to authority and with each other. For the group to survive this tension and grow, we need to understand that such behaviors affirm the strength and vitality of the group. After settling the issue of ownership, the group can proceed to Stage III, Intimacy, where a high degree of mutual aid is present.

Preparing for the Initial Group Meeting: As I prepared for this meeting I thought about how at least three separate constituencies would be represented: those from MITE who knew me and each other; those from the Parish who knew each other and Father C.; and those like Jim and Kate who knew everyone. I expected that in this open-ended group people would come with multiple agendas, and some would be more "in the know" than others. I knew that for the Library Committee to work, these three constituencies would need to agree on a desired outcome and how to work together towards that end. I also knew that the threat I posed to Father C., whose referent power as a priest enhanced his ability to influence the group, would need to be taken into account and softened. Otherwise the group would become divided around our respective visions of change and jeopardize our ability to develop into a working unit.

Fifteen people attended the first library meeting: 10 were members of Father C.'s parish, the remaining five represented three other parishes. Four, including two from Father C.'s parish, had been involved in other MITE activities.

As individuals entered the room there seemed to be a growing sense of cautious anticipation. Some greeted old friends, others watched and waited. I began the meeting by introducing myself and suggesting that everyone give their name and their church affiliation. I said I was an organizer from MITE which was a group of parishes working together to bring change to Midburg. I said I knew people came to discuss the library. Soon after, Father C. talked about the library that was promised 20 years ago. Hopelessness seemed to be the immediate reaction. Mrs. Luria said that's how business is always done in Midburg. Mr. DeLeon said they never give what they promise. For the next 15-20 minutes there was a free floating discussion. Optimism was countered by discouragement; suggestions were countered by other action plans. Many viewpoints were presented. Participants quickly moved to solutions and immediately became frustrated and overwhelmed with the problem. Discouragement was again evident. I felt they were moving too quickly to solutions without solidifying a group contract. This contract would stipulate the problem and a commitment to work on it. To slow them down, I asked the members what it was they wanted, and why now after 20 years! Kate spoke eloquently about her experience as a literacy volunteer and what it was like to have no space, no heat, and no bookshelves. Others joined in with their hopes that their children could use the library.

In approaching this meeting the organizer understood that the group's major task was to develop a shared definition of work, a common problem, and a shared commitment. By having people introduce themselves and their group affiliations he helped the members become familiar with each other thereby reducing "social distance." Though it might be seductive to quickly develop an action plan he knew that premature consensus may be shallow. Thus, he encouraged people to frame the issues in their own terms, define their shared sense of common purpose and, apart from him, to forge a common bond.

Father C. said the Mayor told him the library could be built by a public/private partnership. This arrangement had been tried many times and had rarely succeeded. I knew this view was an expression of his privileged relationship with the Mayor. The idea needed to be challenged but if I did so the group might split. I invited Kate to tell what she learned in her interviews. Kate took pride in her role as expert informant and said the library director felt the public/private arrangement wouldn't work. Everyone noticed that within this group, even a priest could be questioned by other parishioners.

The public/private partnership prompted many questions. My role was to provide information. If the group was to take action, it would need to advance together with shared knowledge, shared sentiment, and accountability to sustain it in the troubled times ahead.

Pessimism came on the heels of the information . . . there's no money, the unions need money, the City's broke. Change isn't possible! I confronted the pessimism directly by providing facts and figures on the budget surplus. This information was met with silence. Father C. said he didn't want to offend anyone in City government. Despite the early call for action, they were still worried about taking risks. They remained uncertain about what I was asking of them and unconvinced about what I was offering.

I knew a lot was at stake and said that all we were trying to do was to help Midburg do its job. I said that I too would not want to offend anyone. Sensing relief that conflict has been bypassed I refocused the group on what we had established, i.e., a shared vision, a broken promise, money to proceed, and many players who can be tapped. The group members were very attentive; they seemed to be together. I moved in and asked what they thought they could do. My appeal was to the group as a whole. Several suggested a petition. I reminded them that about 10 years ago people collected 6,000 signatures. I could not criticize directly without dampening their leadership so I asked what they thought of the idea, hoping they would engage with each other. They vetoed the petition and agreed that a public meeting would be much more effective. The group was back on track.

The organizer in this excerpt understood the strong ambivalence people feel and their reluctance to act. He also understood that passivity can be countered by a sense that others would risk along with them. Despite earlier agreement about the problem, there was no agreement yet about how to proceed. Agreement on an action plan was critical because it would force people to confront their hesitancy to act and would move them from individual to team players. All recognized that a serious though fragile momentum towards change was developing. The organizer used information as a way of keeping alive some measure of hope and instilling a sense of confidence that they could proceed.

> Just when we were getting our momentum back Father C. threw in that he promised the City we wouldn't do anything for 30 days. There was silence. People looked at me. Side stepping the challenge I said we needed to plan anyway, so the 30 days wouldn't pose a problem. Father C. felt relieved because he asked for my help and we worked on plans for the public meeting and for the next meeting of the Committee.

As momentum for change grew the priest became increasingly scared and again attempted to influence the group toward a more conservative path. His admonitions countered the organizer's call to action and raised question about who would provide the leadership and determine the group's direction. To build a sense of communal ownership and bolster the flagging impulse to act, the organizer provided information and encouraged the group to reflect on all ideas. He identified options so the group could consciously make choices. Nothing was done by default; the group affirmed every decision, strengthening itself in the process. Anticipating the priest's challenges, the organizer turned the issues to the group where they rightly belonged. He avoided the head on confrontation which would surely have lead to the group's demise.

> *Preparing for the Second Meeting:* I felt that at our first meeting, the group had arrived at a shared purpose. People entered talking of "I" and left talking of "we." I felt good about that. In the first meeting they deferred to Father C. and me a great deal and I knew I had to help them own the group more. I imagined that each of us might get challenged during this one. I met with Jim, Sam, Kate and knew that their spirits were high and the group was feeling generally more encouraged. I had three concerns for our second meeting: (1) integrating new members into the group, (2) continuing to side step conflict with Father C., and (3) preparing for the public meeting.

Group Meeting #2: There were 12 people at this second meeting, including two from a new parish. Seven people returned from Father C.'s parish, as well as three from two other churches.

As people entered those who were at the last meeting readily greeted each other. After Father C. finished the prayer I began the meeting with introductions and a recapitulation to bring on board the two new members, to update all on what had transpired in the interim, and to reconfirm decisions made last time.

Father C. then gave an update on the public/private partnership. I was surprised how strongly members stated their view that the library had to be a public venture. I remember thinking that they were acting as a group in their challenge of Father C. I said I knew some public/private partnerships worked, but given Midburg's history I didn't think it could work here.

One of the new people asked about the budget surplus and Father C. quoted a figure from the newspaper. I knew that information was wrong. Though I didn't want to challenge him, I couldn't let the group act on misinformation. I said I thought it might be better to use the City's figures and took out copies of a data sheet the City had provided. Father C. didn't protest. He, like everyone else, took the sheet.

A second conflict emerged when Mrs. Lazlo asked about inviting county legislators. I quickly reviewed the role of the county, state, and federal government in the library and suggested they really had none. I asked the group whether they thought the county legislators should be invited. Jim and Kate supported my position. Everyone else said o.k.

With a sense of relief, the group began to plan the specifics of the public meeting. I suggested we think together about what might arise and what the politicians might say. Though people were shy at first, we had some fun role playing the meeting. As they tried on the issue and their role for size, their resolve was strengthened. Ms. Sanchez said they wanted the library right away. How soon was right away, I asked. I knew that the more specific they were, the clearer they would be, and the better the chance for change.

I presented a draft resolution to move the group along. Immediately, Jim clarified it. Because he was respected by many in the group, I considered this challenge to me as the "ultimate" one. My accepting his amendment made our relationship stronger, thereby building the group as a whole.

In this excerpt there are three incidents in which members challenge each other or the organizer. These challenges to the formal and informal authority suggest the group was engaged in Stage II Power and Control, wherein issues of ownership are most important. For the group to develop further, the members had to feel increased collective ownership of the group. When Father C. and the organizer accepted the will of the group, the group as a whole become stronger. When the organizer mediated conflict he facilitated the group's moving on in its work. Having successfully dealt with all three conflicts the original agreement is reconfirmed and work can move on.

After these series of challenges the work of the group really moved forward. I asked them to report to the group as a whole so the entire group would know that whatever was done outside the group had to be approved by the group as a whole. The members moved on to planning the meeting—how it would be billed, who would speak and in what order, when the requests will be presented. Without prompting people began taking roles. Kate said she wanted to present the problem; Jim would present the requests. Luis volunteered to chair. Lucy presented the flyer she drafted for approval and Esther offered to add graphics and to distribute 1000 flyers to local buildings and churches. Esther raised the petition idea again but accepted the will of the group when it rejected it.

The group is demonstrating the mutual aid which characterizes Stage III Intimacy. Norms of mutual aid developed quickly. The group handled difference and potential conflict easily. Having asserted their own leadership and temporarily put aside issues of power and control, the members' energy was directed towards task accomplishment.

Father C. asked the group's approval of a letter he wanted to send to area churches and synagogues. The members seemed struck that even he demonstrated his accountability to the group. They seem pleased with themselves as they confirm the agenda for the final planning meeting before the public hearing.

This group moved very far along and, by the end of the meeting the group as a whole showed real esprit de corps. Once the formal and informal leaders were challenged and members had differed with each other, mutual aid increased dramatically. This happens often, in some form or another, as a precondition for moving into Stage III, intimacy. The organizer had been skillful in mediating conflict, in responding to challenges, and in urging the group to assert its leadership. Task accomplishment was high and members seemed pleased with themselves.

Preparing for the Third Meeting: I felt good going into this meeting and realized a lot had been achieved. I also knew there was a good deal of work to do before the community meeting. I expected people to come eager to work.

Present: There were 37 people: 17 had previously attended the Library Committee meetings, seven were active in MITE, and 15 were newcomers who had no previous contact with the Library Committee or MITE. Of the newcomers eight were from Father C.'s parish, and the remaining five were brought by friends in other churches. Sam Jones, MITE'S assertive Afro-American chairperson and Carmen Gomez, MITE's respected Latino secretary-treasurer were present.

We again began with introductions and newcomers were introduced to oldtimers. The mood was light and there was anticipation and eagerness in the air.

After the prayer Father C. said there was no word on the public/private partnership and therefore he would not raise it at the public meeting. The members allowed themselves a visible sigh of relief. I wasn't surprised when Sam directly confronted the priest, saying it wouldn't work anyway. He made it clear he was willing to bring photos of the many abandoned public/

private projects in case the Mayor pushed his agenda. Everyone watched. Father C., immediately fearing a confrontation with the City Council, reminded everyone that he didn't want any conflict. This was a tense moment. Feeling the group was strong enough now to cope with some diversity, I said I didn't think we could totally avoid conflict. To win there must be some conflict. No one supported Father C. and Sam continued with updated information the group needed.

Sam and Carmen have worked with the organizer in other MITE efforts and they met prior to this meeting. Their prior experience and "inside" information allowed them to enter the group with a level of confidence and knowledge greater than that of other group members present at previous meetings. Sam's assertive challenge to the priest's pessimism, would have, at an earlier time, been met with uneasiness on the part of the members. At this point, however, the group is strong enough to tolerate open conflict and to air differences. The group as a whole has developed a culture which can now sustain such an assertive stance. The strength of the group as a whole provided individual members and the organizer with enough comfort and confidence to openly challenge a priest. As the formal leader, this priest understood that ownership of the group was in the members' hands.

Having successfully met this challenge to its leadership, the group immediately moved to task accomplishment. The members became busy making plans for the meeting, e.g., timing, arrangements, invitations, and division of labor. Mrs. Armon, there for the first time, said she thought it was disrespectful to limit the time of speakers. They were important people and we shouldn't anger them. Several members, explaining the group's position, confirmed their decision about how to approach the public officials. Sister Mary's request for breaks in the program was granted, more in deference to her position than to the need for it.

The pace of the meeting was quick. I found myself saying little. Carmen offered to coordinate refreshments and said that she would get friends to join. Seating arrangements, introductions, how to handle people who want to speak from the floor, timekeeping and a myriad of other details were handled directly from member to member. I was impressed at how they spoke with each other and no longer had to go through me.

Father C. said he was concerned about the turnout. The members said they weren't worried; they would do the best they could and they thought that would be fine. It pleased me that the members could speak directly to Father C. and I no longer had to counter his pessimism.

Having successfully handled issues of power and control in the second meeting, and having established a culture of mutual aid directed at task accomplishment, the members could withstand challenges to their ownership from Father C. and from new members. The group could absorb new people while continuing to progress in its tasks. After seven months of work, the group has successfully negotiated with the Mayor and City Council to put architectural and engineering planning funds for the library in the City's current operating budget, and to begin construction next year.

CONCLUSION

Community organizers are intrinsically concerned about building a working group. People may not initially join, may leave instead of remain, members' goals may be preempted by the organizer, and the group may disintegrate instead of develop. Some working knowledge about how groups come together and develop is indispensable if one is to avoid such disagreeable consequences. It is, for example, important to understand the inevitability of ambivalence about joining and participating and the normative concerns of members about power and control. Organizers are likely to be more skillful in mitigating ambivalence and managing issues of power and control if they have some knowledge of group theory and practice. It is plainly wiser to allow for ambivalence and work patiently with it; to support expressions of hope; to sustain a belief in change by providing information about issues and ways to resolve them and finally, to strengthen the impulse to action and risk taking. Equally important are the organizer's ability to help the group move beyond concerns with ownership and to hear their challenges as positive affirmations of involvement.

NOTES

1. For discussions of the importance of organization building, see for instance, Delgado, G., *Organizing the Movement: The Roots and Growth of ACORN*, Phila.: Temple University Press, 1986, Twelvetress, A., *Democracy and the Neighborhood*, London: National Federation of Community Organizations, 1985, 27-37; Staples, L., *Roots to Power*, NY: Praeger Press, 1984, 14-17; Kahn, S., *Organizing: A Guide for Grassroots Leaders*, NY: McGraw-Hill, 1982, 57-77; Brager and Specht, *Community Organizing*, NY: Columbia University Press, 1973, 142-167; Alinsky, *Reveille for Radicals* NY: Vintage Books, 1969, 53-63.

2. Mondros and Wilson, "Staying Alive: Selecting, Training, and Sustaining Community Organizers," *Administration in Social Work*, Vol. 14, No. 2, 1990.

3. For a discussion of phases of work in groups, see W. Schwartz (1971) "On the Use of Groups in Social Work Practice," In W. Schwartz and S. Zalba (Eds.), *The Practice of Group Work*, NY: Columbia University Press, 3-24.

4. For a discussion about people's reasons for inaction see Bicklen, D., *Community Organizing: Theory and Practice*, Englewood Cliffs, N.J.: Prentice-Hall, Inc., 1983, 21-29.

5. T. Berman-Rossi (Forthcoming) "Empowering Groups Through Understanding Stages of Group Development," *Social Work with Groups* and T. Berman-Rossi (Forthcoming) "The Tasks and Skills of the Social Worker Across Stages of Group Development," *Social Work with Groups*.

6. For a fuller discussion of the Stages of Group Development Literature, see for instance: Bennis, W. and H. Shephard. (1956) "A Theory of Group Development," *Human Relations*. Vol 9, 415-457; Chin, R. (1969) "The Utility of Systems Models and Developmental Models for Practitioners," In W. Bennis, K. Benne, and R. Chin (Eds.) *The Planning of Change*. (2nd ed.) N.Y.: Holt, Rinehart and Winston; Garland, J., H. Jones, and R. Kolodney, (1965) "A Model for Stages of Group Development in Social Work Groups," In S. Bernstein (ed.) *Explorations in Group Work: Essays in Theory and Practice*, Boston: Boston University School of Social Work, and M. Galinsky and J. Schopler (1989), "Developmental Patterns in Open-Ended Groups," *Social Work with Groups*, 12(2), 99-114.

7. See for instance, Mondros, J. and McGuffin, N., *Yonkers: A Tale of Two Cities, Casebook for Social Workers*, NY: The Haworth Press, Inc. 1991 and Staples, *Op. Cit.*

8. Henderson, P. and Thomas, D. *Skills in Neighborhood Work*, London: Allen and Unwin, 1987, 174-190.

9. Garland, Jones, and Kolodney, *Op. Cit.*

BOOK REVIEWS

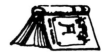

EFFECTIVE SOCIAL ACTION BY COMMUNITY GROUPS. *Alvin Zander. San Francisco: Jossey-Bass Publishers. 1990. 245 pages.*

This book aims to describe how community groups for social change get started, choose objectives, select methods or strategies, and respond to the influence of those whose help they desire. The book is addressed to researchers who are encouraged to further test the ideas presented. More importantly, it is addressed to "agents of change," including reformers, innovators, consultants as well as social workers, who want to create and manage effective social action organizations. The types of organizations Alvin Zander is interested in are social movements, improvement associations, pressure groups, citizen participation groups, citizen action groups, and community groups for social action.

Dr. Zander, now retired, was director of the Research Center for Group Dynamics at the University of Michigan from 1948 to 1980. Many group workers will recall that we gained our first knowledge about group dynamics from the readings he edited with his colleague, Dorwin Cartwright.[1]

This present book is reminiscent of one by Jack Rothman,[2] in which he developed action principles for organizing social change activities from social science research. Zander follows suit giving us sixteen generalizations including hypotheses on why individuals form activist groups, what their motives are, the willingness of members to participate in change activities, how leadership is exercised, how strategies are chosen, the effectiveness of various permissive and pressuring strategies, and what kinds of resistance and counter-influence can be expected from targeted persons and organizations. Yet where Rothman arrives at his principles from systematic meta-analytic techniques, Zander draws his generalizations less systematically and only partly from the social science literature. He also draws on his own experiences and personal observations of social change groups. Being a good scholar, he warns us that many of his generalizations are opinions, albeit "mildly informed ones," and thus open to question.

This book has a number of strengths. The book is clearly written and readable. Although it has no explicit theoretical framework, the book is coherent in its implicit use of a social learning/exchange theory perspective. It is also coherent in its organization; after describing a typology of groups each generalization is presented and discussed in depth. The central contribution of the book is its analysis of the psychology of group participation, influence and counterinfluence. Social workers will want to read the book largely for this analysis.

For this reviewer, the book has one major limitation. It lacks a theory of society, a larger context in which to understand the tensions that give rise to the need for social action, the emergence of group interests, and the dynamics of success and failure. The kind of framework, for instance, that Ralf Dahrendorf[3] offered in writing about social structure, group interests, and conflict groups. Social action for Zander refers as equally to the desire to organize a musical band as it does to organizing on behalf of civil rights and justice. His examples of change, while generally progressive, may as equally be conservative as radical or as politically neutral. His understanding of society is one in which all people seem to have equal opportunity to promote their interests if they can motivate themselves and use the correct strategies. It is not a world of class conflict, of race, gender and age stratification, of advantage and disadvantage, nor of different access to power, resources and the means of control. In short, this reviewer believes that generalizations about the structure and dynamics of society must be the starting point for proposing generalizations about the typology of action groups and the psychology of group participation and influence.

John F. Longres
Professor of Social Work
University of Wisconsin-Madison,
School of Social Work

NOTES

1. Cartwright, D., & A. Zander (Eds.) 1968. *Group Dynamics*. 3rd ed. New York: Harper & Row.
2. Rothman, J. 1974. *Planning and Organizing for Social Change*. New York, N.Y.: Columbia University Press.
3. Dahrendorf, R. 1959. *Class and Class Conflict in Industrial Society*. Palo Alto: Stanford University Press.

GROUP WORK: A HUMANISTIC APPROACH. Urania Glassman and Len Kates. *Newbury Park, CA: Sage. 1990, 294 pages, $31.32 hardback, also in paper.*

Urania Glassman and Len Kates have drawn on their rich experience in practice and teaching to produce a very useful extension of the humanistic group work approach. They not only affirm the viability of the humanistic tradition in group work, but they also identify eight critical values, specify the democratic norms that operationalize these values, and then translate these values and norms into specific practitioner behaviors that are geared toward empowering persons who are victimized. The basic theme of this book is how to develop a culture that shapes cooperative exchange. The emphasis is on the way group work practitioners use humanistic and democratic group processes to simultaneously change inner and interpersonal selves through the group experience. Through the concept of externality, the authors also recognize the importance of the surrounding world to the group experience.

The authors of this book elaborate on what they see as the unique feature of the humanistic approach, the explicit development of the democratic group form or mutual aid system combined with the actualization of group purpose. Glassman and Kates frame their discussion in terms of two major dimensions of practice: humanistic values and democratic norms and stages of group development. They provide a framework for group development, offer specific techniques for promoting the development of groups and the accomplishment of member goals, and describe a wide array of practice examples. Although, as the authors acknowledge, the humanistic approach may not be appropriate for all groups, this book should prompt all group leaders to examine the value premises underlying their interventions.

Glassman and Kates offer a new perspective on the way groups develop. Their schema emphasizes the sequential themes which appear in the humanistic approach. Their eight stages, ranging from "We're not in charge" to "This isn't good anymore" to "Just a little longer," represent a synthesis and expansion of ideas from the Boston School and the T group conceptions of group development. For each of these stages they explore the relevant values and norms and delineate practitioner issues and actions. In keeping with the humanistic tradition, group development is presented in terms of members' subjective response to the evolving system. Further, the authors emphasize the importance of developing supportive systems before groups can actualize their purposes.

This model of humanistic group work seems particularly relevant considering the current proliferation of support groups. In these groups people join together to share common problems and issues and assume responsibility for the conduct of the group. The development of a mutual aid system often characterizes the purpose of the group as well as its style of interaction. Practitioners who lead support groups, those who provide consultation to member run groups, or those who are themselves members of such groups, will find the framework and the techniques presented in this book especially helpful.

The book provides the reader with specific techniques for shaping group culture. This is a useful addition, since most literature on group practice emphasizes the important role of norms in influencing group behavior, but gives only limited consideration to how to guide the group in its development of group standards and rules. The authors specify practitioner behavior needed to operationalize values and norms throughout the stages of group life. Further, the authors place the techniques identified within the framework of the dual purposes of group work, the promotion of the mutual aid system and the actualization of purpose. They propose techniques for each purpose, as well as those which have a dual focus. They use handy labels for each technique which serve to remind the practitioner of their appropriate application, e.g., group mending, taking stock. These techniques are helpful for those who want to understand how the worker intervenes or enters into the life of the group and for those who have acted intuitively and can benefit from concepts which will describe their behavior and enable them to generalize this behavior to their future practice.

The book is outstanding in terms of the examples the authors use to illustrate major ideas, worker roles and member relationships. A rich and varied array of group situations is presented. The reader will gain a practical understanding of the way in which this group model is employed with a diversity of populations, problems and settings. Throughout the book Glassman and Kates provide a framework for operationalizing professional commitments to values. They give a vivid sense of how the social worker joins with the group to create a complex and dynamic system. No matter what practice theory one espouses, this book offers sensitive descriptions of the flow of group process, member interactions, and practitioner responses.

The authors base their model on an experiential, existential, and philosophical foundation. Their focus is on the interaction between the group leader and the group members, on the unfolding of the relationship, and on the values that should guide interaction. They clearly state the parameters of their approach and point to the kinds of practice for which this model will not be useful, such as psychoeducational groups and leader structured groups. Readers of this book should be aware of the stated limitation. The authors give a clear message of what they believe to be the appropriate interventions, but they do not discuss alternatives to the interventions they recommend within the framework of the approach of democratic decision-making. Thus, readers who draw on other conceptual models of group work to guide their practice with groups may find that they would operationalize humanistic values through different interventions than those suggested by Glassman and Kates. At times, a more directive and planful stance may be a preferred mode and more active intervention may be needed. The authors do not deny or denigrate such means of approaching practice, but neither do they deal with them.

The book also is limited by the lack of attention to the systematic evaluation of group work practice. While the authors stress the need for ongoing assessment throughout the life of the group in relation to the development of the democratic mutual aid system and the actualization of purposes, they do not provide a framework for evaluation. Their discussion of psychosocial parameters to assess member behavior in the group is helpful in understanding group interaction but does not promote the examination of the achievement of either process or outcome-oriented objectives. Currently, there is widespread recognition in the social work profession that the evaluation of practice is critical for knowledge building and the advancement of practice. Further work on the humanistic approach should address the need for evaluation. In addition, more consideration of the social science and practice literature based on empirical study of group phenomena would enhance the foundations of humanistic group work practice.

The humanistic approach detailed by Glassman and Kates can either serve as a primary framework for practice or provide a useful supplement to other models. The model focuses to a great extent on how to build an interactive system of members helping members. This viewpoint is important even if the meetings are highly structured to carry out a particular educational or treatment objective. Further, the model provides a sense of the respectful, caring and personal relationship that should characterize the encounter between the social group worker and the group members. It is crucial that those who are engaged in group work practice be familiar with a range of options for leadership behavior. The humanistic model offers a useful perspective and those who lead groups would be advised to read it carefully and to extract the wisdom it contains for working with groups.

Maeda J. Galinsky, MSW, PhD, Professor
Janice H. Schopler, MSW, PhD, Associate Professor
School of Social Work
University of North Carolina at Chapel Hill

Index